About the authors

Roy Jennings is Emeritus Professor in the Section of Infection and Immunity, Division of Genomic Medicine at the University of Sheffield. He graduated in microbiology from the University of Birmingham in 1960, gaining his PhD in 1967 at the University of the West Indies by working on respiratory viral infections. On returning to the UK, he spent five years as a Lecturer in Virology in the Department of Microbiology at the University of Leeds before moving to the Department of Medical Microbiology at the University of Sheffield Medical School. He was Professor of Virology and Head of Department from 1993 to 1999. His research work has been primarily concerned with the disease of influenza, the influenza viruses and their control. He has published over 90 scientific papers on these topics.

Robert C Read is a Reader in Infectious Diseases in the Section of Infection and Immunity, Division of Molecular and Genetic Medicine at the University of Sheffield Medical School, and Honorary Consultant Physician to the Sheffield Teaching Hospitals. He received his medical undergraduate training at the University of Sheffield, and has postgraduate training experience in Leeds, Bristol, London, Nottingham and San Francisco. His research interests include the pathogenesis and prevention of severe infections of the respiratory tract, including influenza.

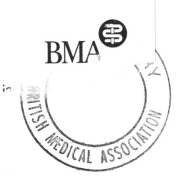

Influenza

in Practice

Roy Jennings

Emeritus Professor, Section of Infection and
Immunity, Division of Genomic Medicine,
University of Sheffield, UK

Robert C Read

Reader in Infectious Diseases, Section of
Infection and Immunity, Division of
Molecular and Genetic Medicine, University
of Sheffield Medical School, UK

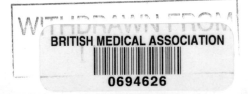

1 Wimpole Street, London W1G 0AE, UK
207 E Westminster Road, Lake Forest, IL 60045, USA
http://www.rsm.ac.uk

British Library Cataloguing in Publication Data
A catalogue record for this book is available from the British Library

ISBN 1-85315-514-4
ISSN 1473-6845

Phototypeset by Phoenix Photosetting, Chatham, Kent
Printed in Europe by the Alden Group, Oxford

Preface

Influenza is currently under the spotlight for several reasons. In the modern era where rapid and relatively easy global travel is commonplace, the spread of infectious diseases, particularly those involving transmission via the respiratory tract, represents a very real and almost annual threat to communities worldwide. Among the high-density population in the UK, recent epidemics of influenza have caused widespread morbidity together with extensive levels of mortality in certain risk groups. These widespread outbreaks have sometimes been accompanied by disruption to essential health care and other services. The epidemics and outbreaks of influenza have also given rise to considerable adverse publicity, largely directed at the government of the time and its policies, or lack of them, for dealing with such eventualities. The fact that such illness, death and disruption can still occur in a modern society in spite of the availability of both a vaccine against the disease and an extensive surveillance network to monitor the appearance and spread of influenza virus strains, serves only to illustrate the magnitude of the problem.

However, over recent years, a number of important scientific advances in man's ongoing battle with the influenza virus and the disease it causes have given rise to optimism that the annual impact of the disease may be reduced in the near future. Progress in understanding both the epidemiology of influenza and its transmission to humans, and the immune mechanisms that underlie the control of the infection, is fuelling both the current development of novel vaccines, as well as the recognition that there could be more effective methods of delivery for these preparations than the conventional intramuscular route. In addition, the past five years have witnessed the advent of a number of drugs that are able to reduce the symptoms of influenza, provided they are administered early enough in the infection.

This book, primarily aimed at medical practitioners working in either the general community or industrial- or company-based practices, should also be found useful by hospital-based consultants, junior doctors, nursing staff and other individuals connected with the healthcare profession. Besides reviewing and updating the biological characteristics of the influenza viruses, the book explains the epidemiological and immune mechanisms that have important roles in, and form the background to, the pathogenesis of influenza infection. Two chapters describe the clinical features of influenza as it presents in different population groups. The current situation with respect to the use of vaccines for immunization against influenza, and the nature and rationale behind the recent development of the anti-influenza drugs, constitute a further two chapters. The final chapter is concerned with the management of influenza in general practice.

Roy Jennings
Robert C Read
January 2002

Contents

Introduction

The illness that we call influenza, and the viruses responsible for causing this infection, probably date back to antiquity. The 'Great Plague' of Athens, dating to about 430–437 BC, may well have been influenza; Thucydides recorded that it killed several thousands of the city's inhabitants including the great Athenian general and leader Pericles. Down through the centuries other descriptions also suggest widespread influenza infections and epidemics erupting from time to time, for example the 'English Sweat' of 1485 and 1551. In the modern era it was the devastating pandemic of 1918 – 'Spanish' or 'swine' influenza – that first brought the disease to worldwide public notice. Over the past few years, outbreaks or epidemics of influenza, of greater or lesser severity, seem to have become a regular feature of life in the UK almost every winter. There is an increased awareness of the medical and economic burdens that have to be shouldered by the community to meet and control infection by these viruses. Influenza infection contributes to a significant annual increase in both morbidity and mortality in the UK during every winter season. It is associated with at least 3000–4000 deaths, primarily in elderly persons suffering from some form of chronic illness. During a substantial epidemic more than 20 000 excess deaths may occur, and the effects may be compounded by severe disruption to essential services.

In spite of the undoubted community-wide effects of influenza epidemics and outbreaks, there are currently grounds for optimism in improving control of the infection. These are due, in part, to the recent development of several new, safe anti-influenza drugs, which have been shown to be efficacious in clinical trials and are now available for use in specific population groups. These novel compounds, which act specifically against the virus, can shorten and ameliorate the clinical symptoms of influenza and also reduce the extent of virus shedding in nasal secretions, thereby showing potential for reducing spread of the virus. Some of these drugs also exhibit some prophylactic potential against influenza virus infection. There is also increasing optimism that progress towards the prevention of influenza through novel vaccination strategies is being made. It is generally agreed that the current commercially available influenza vaccines, although showing a degree of efficacy in reducing morbidity and mortality in certain groups within the population, are less than ideal, particularly in the face of a large-scale epidemic or pandemic associated with a novel Type A strain of virus.

The influenza Type A viruses possess the capacity to undergo consistent genetic variation of their nucleic acid, resulting in regular, indeed almost annual, phenotypic modifications and changes in the protein antigens present on their surface. In turn, such alterations in antigenic structure influence the extent of recognition of these proteins by the immune defences of the host when virus infection takes place. This 'trick' is the main means by which the influenza virus has evaded complete control by vaccination until now, despite the considerable efforts of researchers and clinicians since the initial isolation of the virus in 1933. Over the past decade or so, however, burgeoning molecular biology and genetic engineering technology has led to the development of several novel vaccines, produced through the use of clever and complex molecular and genetic strategies, against many different microbial agents. Some of these vaccines have become commercially available for all or specific population groups. There is currently considerable interest and research into the application of these strategies for the further development of influenza vaccines. These novel approaches have been coupled with the parallel development of methodology that will permit effective delivery of such vaccine preparations into the respiratory tract of the human host – the most appropriate site for preventing influenza virus infection. These researches, which have been accompanied by an increased understanding of the nature of the immune mechanisms operating against influenza viruses in the human respiratory tract, suggest that a new generation of such vaccines may become a reality within the next three to five years.

> There is an increased awareness of the medical and economic burdens that are shouldered by the community to meet and control infection by influenza viruses

This book provides an overview of the virological and clinical aspects of influenza. It includes chapters devoted to the pathogenesis of the disease and the interaction of the viruses with host tissues and immune defences, the epidemiology of the infection and its relevance and impact on those groups at greatest risk from the disease, and the current situation with regard to control and treatment of the infection through vaccines and anti-influenza drugs.

Further reading

Langmuir AD, Worthen TD, Solomon J *et al*. The Thucydides syndrome. A new hypothesis for the cause of the plague of Athens. *N Engl J Med* 1985; **313**: 1027–30.

1. Nature of the influenza viruses

Structure
Growth and replication
Variability
Nomenclature
Influenza viruses in non-human
    species
Type B and C influenza viruses

Influenza viruses are members of the family Orthomyxoviridae, which incorporates three virus types: the influenza Types A, B and C. The basis of the difference between these virus types lies in the molecular nature of a major internal protein, the ribonucleoprotein (RNP), which surrounds the ribonucleic acid (RNA) gene segments.

- The Type A and B influenza viruses contain eight RNA gene segments.
- The Type C influenza virus contains only seven RNA gene segments.

The RNA gene segments of the Type A and B viruses code for 11 viral proteins, three of which are located on the surface of the mature virus particle (virion). Seven of the remaining proteins are located in the virion interior and have multiple functions concerned with:

- virion integrity
- protection of the viral RNA
- translocation of virion components within the host cell
- replication, packaging, assembly and maturation of the virus in the host cell.

Four of these internal proteins, the RNP protein itself plus the three P proteins that make up the polymerase enzyme of the virus, form the structure of the viral nucleocapsid. Functionally, these proteins form the transcriptase complex. They act in concert and are instrumental in 'kick-starting' virus replication within the infected host cell. Another protein, recently termed the 'nuclear export protein', appears to have the major function of ensuring proper egress of progeny viral nucleocapsids from the host cell nucleus. One other protein, the non-structural protein NS1, which also contributes to virus replication and the intracellular translocation of virion components, is expressed from the viral genome only in the infected host cell. It has not been found in the mature virus particles.

There are three types of influenza virus: Type A, Type B and Type C

Structure

The basic structure of the influenza virus consists of a central core or 'nucleocapsid' containing most of the internal proteins and the viral RNA segments (Figure 1.1). External to the nucleocapsid, but closely associated and integral with it, is a major structural protein of the virus. This matrix (M1) protein is primarily responsible for virion integrity. The M1 protein also interacts with the structure external to it – the lipid envelope of the virus, which carries three important viral glycoproteins. The function of the glycoproteins is in the entry and exit of the virus in the host cell. These glycoproteins project through the lipid envelope and appear as 'spikes' in electron micrographs. The lipids in the envelope of the influenza virus are derived from the host cell. This is because the virus is assembled at and emerges through the cell membrane on completion of its replication cycle.

Mature extracellular influenza virus particles are normally approximately spherical, ranging in size from about 90 to 120 nm in diameter (Figure 1.2).

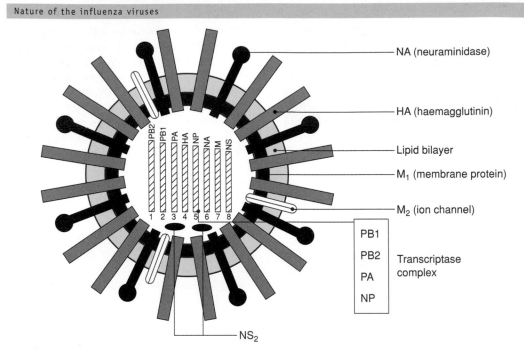

Figure 1.1

Schematic representation of an influenza virus particle. [Reproduced from De Jong JC, Rimmelzwaan CF, Fouchier RA, Osterhaus AD. Influenza virus: a master of metamorphosis. *J Infect* 2000; **40**: 218–28. With kind permission of the publisher WB Saunders]

Growth and replication

The replication cycle of the virus starts with attachment of the virus to specific receptors on susceptible host cells. In humans, these are usually epithelial cells lining the respiratory passages. These receptors have been identified as the terminal sialic (neuraminic) acid residues on the oligosaccharide side-chains of susceptible cells.

The virus then penetrates the host cell inside an endocytic vesicle where it is 'uncoated' – the lipid envelope and matrix protein of the particle are degraded by host cell processes. These processes include a marked reduction in the pH inside the endocytic vesicle. The lowered pH also triggers a structural change in the surface haemagglutinin (HA) protein antigen of the virus and exposes the viral nucleocapsid. The nucleocapsid, which contains the viral RNA and several viral proteins with enzymatic functions concerned with viral replication, is unaffected

by the low pH. It remains intact, and is released into the cell cytoplasm once the vesicle undergoes natural degradation. The nucleocapsid then migrates to the nucleus of the host cell.

In the nucleus, the viral RNA and the associated viral enzymes direct the formation of messenger RNA for the manufacture of progeny viral proteins in the cell cytoplasm, and progeny viral RNA in the nucleus. Following the relocation of several of these progeny molecules into the nucleus of the host cell and the formation of progeny nucleocapsids, the latter migrate to the cell surface where they accumulate just beneath the host cell membrane. Other progeny viral molecules, the HA and neuraminidase (NA) in particular, migrate through the cell cytoplasm without prior relocation to the nucleus. They are inserted into the host cell membrane where they project into the surrounding microenvironment. At this point, and under the direction of the M1 protein, maturation of the progeny

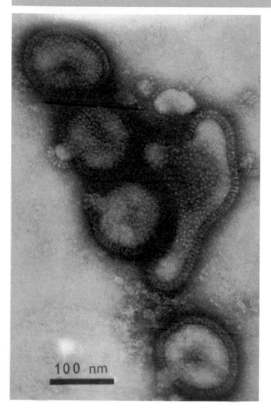

Figure 1.2
Electron micrograph of influenza virus particles.
[Reproduced from Emond RTD, Rowland HAK, Welsby PD. *A colour atlas of infectious diseases*. 3rd edn. London: Wolfe, 1995. With kind permission from Times Mirror International Publishers Ltd.]

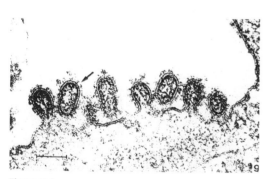

Figure 1.3
Electron micrograph showing influenza virus particles being released from an infected cell by the 'budding' process. Stained with uranyl acetate and lead citrate (x 100 000).

nucleocapsids and assembly with progeny viral surface proteins embedded in the cell membrane takes place. Finally, 'budding' and release of the mature progeny virions occurs by a process termed exocytosis (Figure 1.3). The arrow indicates the surface protein antigen 'spikes' on one of the virus particles. These progeny virions may now infect other, neighbouring, susceptible cells and be shed from the body in the respiratory secretions.

Variability

Although morphologically similar, influenza virus Types A, B and C exhibit different patterns of epidemiological and clinical behaviour. The Type A viruses are associated with most of the widespread influenza epidemics, and are the sole cause of the occasional global pandemics. They have the greatest propensity to cause severe infection and also predispose to secondary bacterial pneumonia in certain groups of the population. The two most abundant surface glycoproteins of the Type A influenza viruses also show the greatest extent of variability, undergoing subtle, minor changes in structure almost annually. These surface proteins, HA and NA, are important as targets for the immune defences in controlling influenza virus infection. The HA glycoprotein is approximately eight times more abundant on the surface of the virus particle than the NA. The minor changes in the structure of these glycoproteins are primarily the consequence of point mutations in the viral RNA genes coding for them. These probably arise because of the absence of a proofreading mechanism to correct mistakes occurring as the virus nucleic acid replicates inside the host cell. This ongoing variability of the Type A virus surface proteins is known as 'antigenic drift'. It is a major reason for their success in evading human immune defence mechanisms and causing frequent outbreaks and epidemics.

> Most influenza epidemics are associated with Type A viruses

Figure 1.4 illustrates the regular outbreaks in the UK caused by the influenza viruses over a 12-year period as a consequence of this antigenic drift.

> The Type A viruses are associated with most influenza epidemics and are the sole cause of the occasional global pandemics. They can cause severe infection, and also predispose to secondary bacterial pneumonia in certain people. They undergo subtle, minor changes in structure almost annually

Nomenclature

The nomenclature of the influenza viruses that infect humans is derived from four components:

- the virus type (A or B)
- the place where the virus was initially isolated, for example Beijing in China
- the sequential number of the isolate as designated by the World Health Organization Influenza Surveillance Network
- the year of isolation.

Thus A/Beijing/32/92 is a Type A virus isolated in Beijing in 1992.

Influenza viruses in non-human species

Several mammalian and avian species are hosts to Type A influenza viruses that bear genetically similar, yet antigenically different versions of the same surface HA and NA proteins as those present on the human Type A viruses. Wild avian species are primary reservoirs for the influenza Type A viruses. Very occasionally humans become infected with a virus bearing HA and/or NA antigens derived from non-human sources. These are essentially novel to humans, and this can give rise to a localized outbreak that may develop into a worldwide influenza pandemic. This is because the HA and/or NA surface antigens of such viruses are not initially recognized by the specific human host defence mechanisms. Because the viruses meet with little or no established resistance, they can spread relatively easily in the human species.

> When humans are infected by a novel virus with a non-human origin, a localized outbreak may occur which could turn into a worldwide pandemic

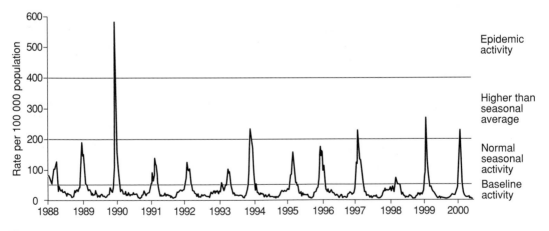

Figure 1.4
Weekly consultation rates for influenza and influenza-like illness. Weekly Returns Service of the Royal College of General Practitioners, 1988–2000. [Adapted from Fleming DM. The contributions of influenza to combined acute respiratory infections, hospital admissions, and deaths in winter. *Commun Dis Public Health* 2000; **3**: 32–8. With kind permission of the PHLS Communicable Disease Surveillance Centre ©PHLS.]

A recent example of this occurred in Hong Kong in 1997, with the infection of humans with an avian influenza virus. Fortunately this small (but nevertheless severe) outbreak was contained and remained localized, with no further spread and no establishment of the virus in humans.

Type B and C influenza viruses

In general, the Type B influenza viruses cause milder illnesses than the Type A viruses. Nevertheless, infection with a Type B virus can range from an illness accompanied by no more than common cold-like symptoms to typical, severe influenza. Symptomatic Type B influenza virus infections are more common in children than in adults. Infections of adults with Type B virus are more often mild or asymptomatic (although occasional severe disease does occur). The frequency of infections with Type B influenza viruses requiring hospitalization is only about one-quarter of that for the Type A viruses.

Although its structure and organization are similar to the Type A influenza viruses, the Type B influenza virus has limited variation in the genes coding for its surface HA and NA proteins, and the mutation rate associated with its RNA is lower than that of the Type A viruses (Table 1.1). The lower mutation rate and lack of mammalian or avian reservoir for the Type B influenza viruses means that they represent less of a clinical or epidemiological problem than the Type A viruses.

The Type C influenza virus is associated with only asymptomatic or mild common cold-like illnesses in humans. Both its genome and its protein structure are organized slightly differently from those of the Type A or B

Table 1.1

Nucleotide substitution rates for the haemagglutinin (HA) gene of the Type A and Type B influenza viruses

Influenza virus type	Annual nucleotide substitution rate in the gene coding for the virus HA protein
A	0.40–0.70%
B	0.18–0.20%

Adapted from Smith DB, Inglis SC. *J Gen Virol* 1987; **68**: 2729–40.

viruses, and it undergoes no antigenic variation of its single surface protein.

The influenza viruses have been recorded as causing infections, outbreaks, epidemics and pandemics in humans from ancient times, and the disease has been considered to be one of the last great uncontrolled plagues of humankind. However, recent advances in both chemoprophylaxis and chemotherapy for the infection indicate that some progress is being made in combating this disease.

> Influenza may be considered to be one of the last great uncontrolled plagues of humankind

Further reading

Ellis J, Joseph C, Zambon M. Fifty years of influenza serveillance. *Commun Dis Public Health* 1999; **2**: 81–2.

Ellis J, Zambon M. Strain designation for influenza viruses. *Commun Dis Public Health* 1999; **2**: 157–9.

Potter CW. A history of influenza. *J Appl Microbiol* 2001; **91**: 572–9.

Ruigrok, RWH. Structure of influenza A, B and C viruses. In: Nicholson KG, Webster RG, Hay AJ (eds) *Textbook of Influenza*. Oxford: Blackwell, 1998.

Smith DB, Inglis SC. The mutation rate and variability of eukaryotic viruses: an analytical review. *J Gen Virol* 1987; **68**: 2729–40.

2. Epidemiology

Infection patterns
Antigenic variability in Type A
 viruses
Type A influenza virus activity in non-
 human hosts
Virulence factors
Resistance to infection

Because the influenza viruses possess a lipid envelope, they are relatively labile. They can only survive in an infectious form on inert surfaces outside the human or animal host for short periods of time. Their survival time is also dependent on the presence of accompanying proteinaceous material. Several carefully conducted studies carried out in the 1980s indicated that the half-life of Type A influenza virus particles in saline on an inert surface in the absence of any protein is approximately two–three hours. However, in the presence of high concentrations of protein, the half-life rises to about four–six hours. Because of these findings it is generally believed that most human influenza virus infections are transmitted through the direct transfer of aerosols or droplets carrying the virus from the respiratory tract of one person to that of another.

Most human influenza virus infections are spread through aerosols or droplets carrying the virus

---

Infection patterns

The incubation period for influenza virus infections are:

- Type A virus – three days
- Type B virus – four days.

Virus replication in the respiratory tract of normal adults peaks approximately 48 hours after infection. Progeny virions are shed in nasal secretions and saliva from about one–seven days after infection (Figure 2.1). Children of preschool and school age are major vectors for influenza virus transmission. In these children the virus is shed from day one postinfection and may still be present up to day 13 postinfection.

Antigenic variability in Type A viruses

A major characteristic of the influenza viruses, particularly the Type A viruses, is the antigenic variability of their surface haemagglutinin (HA) and neuraminidase (NA) proteins.

Antigenic drift

Antigenic drift occurs in both the surface proteins, although it is greatest for the HA protein. It is a virtually ongoing process, resulting from spontaneous point mutations occurring in the viral genes coding for these proteins as the virus replicates in the human body. These mutations are manifest at the phenotypic level as distinct alterations in the reactivity of the surface proteins every two–three years. The manifestations are seen only when the accumulated effect of a series of point mutations becomes detectable by laboratory methods. The changes in the surface protein structure of strains recently isolated from humans can be observed in the laboratory through the altered interaction of their HA or NA proteins with specific antibodies to the HA or NA proteins of existing, previously isolated strains.

Most antigenic variation is seen in the HA protein although the NA protein also undergoes antigenic drift

---

The antigenic changes are responsible for the reduced capacity of any pre-existing antibody to previously experienced influenza virus to combine with and hence effectively neutralize

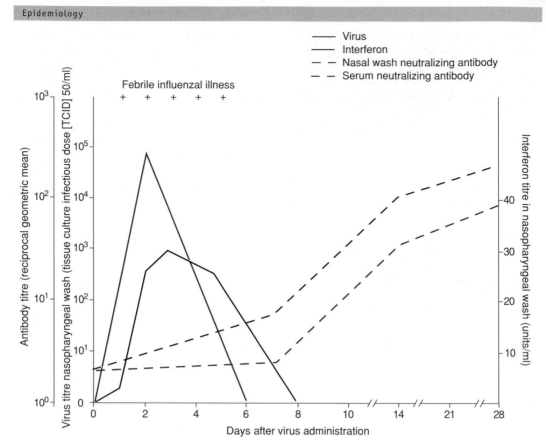

Figure 2.1

Mean patterns of virus titre, serum and nasal wash antibody levels, febrile response and nasal wash interferon levels over time in six seronegative volunteers given $10^{4.0}$ tissue culture infectious doses of wild-type A/Hong Kong/68-like virus intranasally on day 0. [Reproduced from Murphy BR, Webster RG. Orthomyxoviruses. In: Fields BN, Knipe DM, Chanock Rm *et al*. (eds) *Fields' virology*. 2nd edn. Philadelphia, PA: Raven Press, 1990: 1091–152.]

the altered virus strain. The net result of these mutations is an imperfect match between the antigen present on the current virus and the pre-existing antibody induced in response to contact with earlier strains of the virus. This inefficient neutralizing action of the antibody permits a more effective uptake of the modified virus by susceptible cells and therefore a greater probability for the establishment of infection.

Antigenic shift

Laboratory evidence indicates that the 20th century saw five influenza pandemics resulting from the appearance of a Type A virus bearing an HA protein that was essentially novel to the contemporary human population. The best known of these was the pandemic of 1918 – the 'swine' or 'Spanish' influenza epidemic – which reportedly caused in excess of 20 million deaths, primarily in young adults. The most recent, but much less devastating, pandemic occurred in 1977. It saw the reappearance of a virus with an HA protein having similarities to that responsible for the 1918 pandemic, and also to that involved in the pandemic of 1933–34.

Almost all these sudden major changes in the Type A influenza surface antigens initially occurred in China. Several of these 'new' influenza viruses have arisen by genetic reassortment between human and either mammalian or avian influenza viruses bearing different surface proteins. Genetic reassortment has been detected *in vivo* in both humans and animal species. Such reassortment is dependent on the random distribution of the genomic material of two distinct Type A influenza viruses present and undergoing replication in the same cell. In general, the different influenza Type A virus subtypes infect only a single host species. When the occasional cross-species transmission of a subtype occurs, however, genetic reassortment can take place between the transmitted subtype and an influenza Type A virus in the recipient host. This can produce an essentially novel virus bearing surface proteins derived from either parent subtype. Continued replication of this virus in the host can produce further minor modifications of either or both of the surface proteins that may also contribute to its distinct antigenic profile. This virus may now have acquired the capability of infecting a third host, such as humans.

> Each influenza Type A virus subtype usually only infects one host species

Laboratory studies have unequivocally demonstrated that both the 1957 and the 1968 influenza Type A pandemic strains appeared through genetic reassortment. The 1957 'Asian' influenza virus obtained the two genes coding for its HA and NA surface proteins from an avian influenza Type A virus, together with a gene coding for one of its internal proteins. The remaining five genes present in the Asian Type A virus were all derived from the preceding human Type A influenza virus strain, which had been circulating in the human population since 1933–34.

Across all animal species and in humans, there are 15 different HA proteins (H1 to H15) and nine different NA proteins (N1 to N9). To date, only three of the HA proteins (H1, H2 and H3) have been found in those influenza Type A

viruses that are able to infect and become established in humans. In Hong Kong in 1997, however, clear evidence appeared of direct transmission of an influenza virus bearing a non-human HA antigen (the H5 avian influenza virus antigen) from chickens to humans. This occurred despite the fact that avian Type A influenza viruses grow much less efficiently in human cells than in their natural avian host cells. This highly virulent avian Type A virus caused 18 cases of respiratory tract infection in humans, six of them fatal. The patients infected by this virus also suffered from:

- severe haemorrhagic complications
- renal failure.

The severity of the infection in apparently healthy individuals aged 13–60 years was of considerable concern, creating a new awareness of the direct infective potential of avian influenza viruses for humans. Nevertheless, this virus did not spread from one patient to another, and did not therefore become established in humans.

Type A influenza virus activity in non-human hosts

In addition to the recent appearance in humans of influenza Type A viruses bearing the H5 antigen, two uncomplicated human influenza infections with Type A viruses carrying the H9 HA protein previously confined to avian species were reported in 1999. These infections, one in Hong Kong and one in China, were in two children (one and four years old) both of whom recovered fully. In both these instances, humans proved to be 'dead end' hosts and the viruses appeared not to possess the capability to spread from one individual to another and elicit secondary infections.

However, in the catastrophic pandemic of 1918, laboratory and epidemiological evidence indicates that the 'Spanish' or 'swine' influenza virus probably arose by direct transfer of a porcine influenza virus from pigs to humans. The virus subsequently spread very effectively in humans, which on this occasion proved not to be 'dead end' hosts. Direct transfer of influenza Type A viruses from pigs to humans has been documented on several occasions in the past 30 years. This demonstrates that such transmissions can still occur in nature, and pigs may represent the major animal host from which the spread of potentially novel Type A influenza viruses to humans occurs most readily.

Because of the diverse nature of influenza Type A virus receptors on the surface of the cells in their respiratory tract, pigs are easily infected by both avian and human influenza virus Type A subtypes. Pigs have been described as 'mixing vessels' for the generation of novel influenza viruses with potential pandemic capability in humans. The infection of pigs by human viruses also provides opportunities for interactions between human and swine influenza viruses in these animals. Currently there is considerable activity involving epidemics and widespread distribution of the H9N2 influenza Type A virus in both domestic avian species and in pigs. This provides the potential for further instances of spread to humans, and necessitates careful monitoring of the situation.

> The animals from which novel influenza viruses are most readily transmitted to humans are pigs

Since the pandemic of 1977 (known as 'Russian flu' on account of its origin from a laboratory somewhere in the former Soviet Union), two Type A influenza virus subtypes have been circulating among humans worldwide. These subtypes are:

- the H1N1 virus – Russian 'flu
- the H3N2 subtype – which first appeared in the population in 1968 as the cause of the 'Hong Kong' pandemic.

Both viruses have been undergoing antigenic drift since their first appearance in the human population. During the past 24 years, there has been no introduction, spread or establishment of a novel Type A influenza virus on a global scale. The duration and years of prevalence of the various influenza Type A subtypes that have circulated in humans from 1918 to the present time are listed in Table 2.1.

Table 2.1
Subtypes of influenza A viruses found in humans

Influenza A virus subtype	Popular name of virus subtype	Years of prevalence
H1N1 ('swine'-like)	Spanish or swine 'flu	1917–32
H1N1	None	1933–56
H2N2	Asian influenza	1957–67
H3N2	Hong Kong 'flu	1968 to present*
TH1N1	Russian 'flu	1977 to present*

* Influenza A subtype that is currently circulating in humans.

> The current Type A influenza virus subtypes circulating in humans are H3N2 and H1N1

Virulence factors

The inherent virulence of a given strain of Type A influenza virus remains something of an enigma. Well-defined virulence factors are associated with certain Type A influenza viruses that infect domestic poultry, and such highly virulent strains often cause severe mortality and morbidity at considerable economic cost to the poultry industry. But the major virulence factor displayed by the Type A influenza viruses that is associated with the catastrophic epidemics in poultry does not seem to play a significant role in human infection. This property is the cleavability by host enzymes of the linkage site between two sections of the viral HA protein. The reason may be due to:

- the existence of exquisite differences in the nature of the cell receptors on the susceptible human and poultry cells

- differences in the interaction of avian influenza viruses with human host cell enzymes during cell infection and replication.

The inherent virulence of any given virus strain is multifactorial, but one factor that may well contribute to this virulence is the non-sturctural (NS1) protein. Among its roles in the cell biology of the virus, NS1 can effectively inhibit the production by host cells of interferon-inducted antiviral proteins. These proteins have important roles in the cellular control of influenza and of many other viral infections. NS1 can also down-regulate apoptosis (programmed cell death) in cells infected by Type A viruses. The quality or quantity of functional NS1 protein produced during infection by a given strain of influenza Type A virus may therefore influence the capacity of that strain to elicit a more or less severe infection.

There have been one or two reports that both the infection rate and the severity of the associated influenzal illness is greater for the H3N2 strains than for the H1N1 strains in humans. The factors that may play a role in these differences still remain to be determined.

Resistance to infection

Humans acquire resistance to the influenza virus when they have circulating antibodies to the HA and NA surface proteins of the virus. These antigens project through the lipid envelope of the virus and are also expressed at the surface of infected host cells. Infected cells and virions themselves therefore represent important targets for the immune defence mechanisms of the host. In the human (or animal) host, infection with the influenza viruses elicits:

- a humoral immune response
- a cellular immune response.

The humoral element of this immune response is long-lived in the circulation and is specific for the infecting subtype of influenza virus, ie Type A or Type B. In nature, however, the antigenic

drift shown by the Type A influenza viruses means that the full effect of this immunity wanes over time. Its duration at protective levels is dependent on the extent of the antigenic change accumulated by the surface proteins (particularly the HA antigen of the virus). Systemic antibody levels to the HA protein have been correlated with protection against influenza virus infection. The role of local, nasal and respiratory tract antibody is increasingly being recognized as an important contributor to the host's defences against this infection.

Influenza virus-specific cell-mediated immune mechanisms, particularly that due to cytotoxic T-lymphocytes, have a major role in the recovery from infection by the influenza viruses. This is probably through the destruction of influenza virus-infected cells in the respiratory tract. This cellular immune mechanism does not become effective until two or three days after the initial infection. It is more independent of the antigenic variability of the viral surface proteins than the humoral immune response, but is relatively short-lived and lasts for only a few weeks.

> The humoral immune response to an influenza infection is more long lasting than the cell-mediated response, which is only effective for a few weeks

Further reading

Bush RM, Bender CA, Subbarao, K et al. Predicting the evolution of human influenza A. Science 1999; **286**: 1921–25.

De Jong JC, Rimmelzwaan GF, Fouchier RAM, Osterhaus ADME. Influenza virus: A master of metamorphosis. J Infect 2000; **40**: 218–28.

Fields BN, Knipe DM, Chanock RM et al. Fields' Virology, Vol 1, 2nd edn. Philadelphia, PA: Raven Press, 1990: 1103.

Fleming DM. The contribution of influenza to combined acute respiratory infections, hospital admissions, and deaths in winter. Commun Dis Public Health 2000; **3**: 32–8.

Ito T, Couceiro JN, Kelm S et al. Molecular basis for the generation in pigs of influenza A viruses with pandemic potential. J Virol 1998; **72**: 7367–73.

Mortimer P. On being prepared: the influenza Pandemic Plan. *Common Dis Public Health* 2001; **4**: 156–7.

Nguyen-Van-Tam JS. Epidemiology of influenza. In: Nicholson KG, Webster RG, Hay AJ (eds) *Textbook of Influenza*. Oxford: Blackwell, 1998.`

Pickrell J. The 1918 pandemic. Killer flu with a human–pig pedigree. *Science* 2001; **292**: 1041.

Simonsen L. The global impact of influenza on morbidity and mortality. *Vaccine* 1999; **17 Suppl 1**: S3–10.

Webster RG, Bean WJ, Gorman OT *et al.* Evolution and ecology of influenza A viruses. *Microbiol Rev* 1992; **56**: 152–79.

Zhirnov OP, Konakova TE, Wolff T, Klenk HD. NS1 protein of influenza A virus down-regulates apoptosis. *J Virol* 2002; **76**: 1617–25.

3. Pathogenesis

Establishment of infection
Pathogenetic effects
Role of interferon
Role of local host factors
Serum antibody
Protection and clearance

Influenza viruses are transmitted not only via droplet spread in nasal secretions and saliva (expelled particularly during coughing and sneezing), but also during the ordinary daily contact of humans with each other. Particles generated during coughing or sneezing are usually less than 2 mm in diameter. Particles of this size are normally deposited in the lower airways of the lung.

Establishment of infection

The stages of infection with an influenza Type A virus depend on contact of the inhaled virus with susceptible mucosal epithelial cells in the human respiratory tract. This contact allows attachment of the virus to its specific cellular receptors. It is suggested that most successful influenza virus infections are established in the lower respiratory tract. However, this does not necessarily preclude the possibility that a significant number may be initiated in the nasal passages of the upper respiratory tract.

It is also becoming increasingly recognized that an infection is more likely to be successfully established where influenza-specific antibodies, particularly local IgA, are either absent altogether or present at only low levels in the respiratory tract. In the presence of local antibodies, the attachment of influenza virus particles to their specific host cell receptors will be inhibited. The

antibody can also attach to the viral surface proteins, particularly the haemagglutinin (HA), and block the activity of the virus particles.

Most successful influenza virus infections are probably established in the lower respiratory tract

Factors influencing establishment of infection

The closeness of the match between the incoming virus and any existing local antibodies is particularly important when establishing an infection. The presence of local antibodies to Type B influenza, however high their level, will not influence the establishment of a Type A influenza virus infection. Similarly, due to the phenomenon of antigenic drift shown annually by the Type A influenza viruses, the presence of antibodies to a strain of influenza A virus encountered three or four years previously may have a limited effect in preventing establishment of infection by a current Type A strain. Following establishment of the virus, there may be a very transient viraemia, but it is generally not possible to recover virus from the bloodstream of infected individuals. Similarly, there is no unequivocal evidence that the virus can persist or exist in any latent form in the human host.

The ability of the influenza viruses to establish infection in humans will thus be dependent on:

- several nonspecific and virus-specific host factors
- viral factors, such as the quantity of virus inhaled or taken in to the respiratory tract
- the intrinsic virulence of the virus.

The larger the amount of virus taken into the respiratory tract, the greater the chance the virus has of overcoming any local specific, extracellular defence mechanisms (particularly local antibody). It is also more likely that the virus will attach to and penetrate susceptible mucosal columnar epithelial cells. As part of the nonspecific defences of the host, the

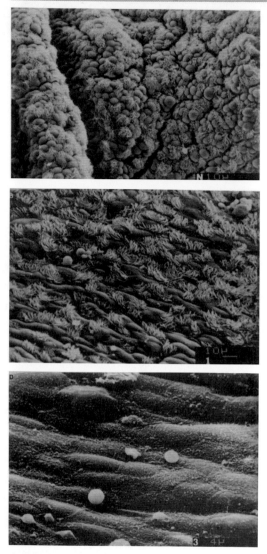

Figure 3.1
Scanning electron micrographs of normal mouse tracheal epithelium [× 1050] (upper panel), mouse tracheal epithelium [× 800] 24 hours after infection with Type A virus showing partial destruction of the ciliated nasal epitheial cells (centre panel), and the same cells [× 2000] 72 hours postinfection, showing complete destruction of the cells (bottom panel). [Reproduced from Ramphal *et al. American Review of Respiratory Diseases* 1979; **120**: 1313–24.]

mucociliary escalator will remove a proportion of the invading virus particles. This is most effective in healthy nonsmoking individuals.

> The ability of influenza virus to establish infection depends on various host factors, the quantity of virus in the respiratory tract and how virulent the particular virus strain is

Pathogenetic effects

The lytic replication cycle of the virus commences as soon as it enters a cell. After about five or six hours, this results in the release of progeny virus particles, which spread gradually to other susceptible cells. In humans this ultimately results in almost total destruction of the ciliated epithelial cells of the respiratory tract. Similar effects can be observed in ferrets and mice – both good models for human influenza virus infection (Figure 3.1). In both the mouse and ferret, regeneration of the ciliated cells is underway by seven to 10 days from the start of infection.

Destruction of epithelial cells

Influenza virus infection in the human nasopharynx results in a loss of the ciliated epithelial cells in this area and also in the trachea (Figure 3.2). These cells are an important element of the human nonspecific respiratory tract defences. A major consequence of their destruction is to pave the way for secondary invasion of the lower respiratory tract by bacteria, such as *Streptococcus pneumoniae*, *Staphylococcus aureus* and *Haemophilus influenzae*. This can lead to severe or even fatal pneumonia, particularly in the elderly and other high-risk groups. Bronchoscopy of individuals with uncomplicated influenza virus infection shows the bronchi, trachea and larynx to be:

- de-ciliated
- oedematous
- acutely inflamed.

The cells are then desquamated.

> Influenza infection results in almost total destruction of the ciliated epithelial cells of the respiratory tract, which paves the way for secondary bacterial infections

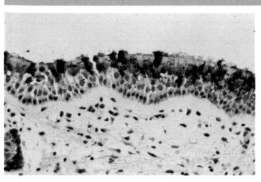

Figure 3.2
Histopathological appearance of human nasopharyngeal explant collected three days after the onset of influenza Type B infection. Stained by an immunoperoxidase method using a polyclonal sheep anti-influenza serum. There is patchy uptake of virus in the epithelial cells, which will ultimately exfoliate.

Role of interferon

Infection of humans by the influenza viruses probably promotes the full repertoire of the immune and non-immune (nonspecific) responses of the host. However, the viruses appear to trigger the interferon response of the host extremely effectively. Moreover, there is a direct correlation between the quantities of interferon released from the host's infected cells and the extent of virus replication. Interferon is first detected in both the upper respiratory tract secretions and the blood of infected individuals when the clinical symptoms of influenza commence. The levels of interferon reach a peak about 24 hours later. The cytokine almost certainly plays an important role in reducing replication and limiting spread of the virus in the respiratory tract of the host.

There has been some evidence to show that the clinical symptoms of influenza, particularly the systemic symptoms of malaise, aching back and joints and high temperature, are associated with high levels of interferon. These symptoms are also possibly associated with other proinflammatory cytokines such as interleukin-6 and tumour necrosis factor. Tumor necrosis factor-α has recently been reported to possess stronger anti-influenza virus activity than other cytokines present in human nasal lavage specimens.

Role of local host factors

Other nonspecific host factors that play a part in the control of influenza virus infection include:

- soluble factors, such as lung surfactants
- sialylglycoproteins
- alveolar macrophages.

All of these can react with or take up influenza virus particles. Such reactions thereby prevent them from attaching to and invading the susceptible columnar epithelial cells of the respiratory tract. Another prime factor in controlling infection by the influenza viruses is the presence at the time of infection of influenza virus-specific local and systemic antibodies.

Local antibody response

During a primary influenza virus infection (ie one occurring in a host who has never experienced infection by an influenza virus in the past), IgA, IgG and IgM antibodies specific for the virus HA antigen can be detected in nasal washings collected 24–48 hours after the onset of symptoms. The IgA antibodies are actively secreted locally. The IgG antibody is almost certainly derived from the transudate that spills into the respiratory tract secretions from the bloodstream as a consequence of the inflammatory changes taking place as the infection progresses. Both IgA and IgG antibodies are capable of neutralizing the virus by preventing its attachment to, or entry into, susceptible columnar epithelial cells. This is done through attaching to the virus particles, thereby blocking the activities of the HA protein, which is the prime mediator of these viral functions.

There is immunological memory for the local IgA response stimulated following a primary (and a secondary) infection. This is specific for the HA and NA antigens present on the surface of the infecting virus. Changes in the antigenic

Table 3.1
Correlation of HA antibody status with infection in groups of volunteers infected with a Type A influenza virus

Antibody status of the group				
Serum antibody	Nasal wash antibody	Total number in group	Number infected	Percentage infected
Absent	Absent	16	10	62
Absent	Present	1	0	0
Present	Absent	12	4	33
Present	Present	6	1	17

[Adapted from Betts RF, Treanor JJ. Approaches to improved influenza vaccinations. *Vaccine* 2000; **18**: 1690–95. With kind permission from Excerpta Medica Inc.]

structure of these proteins through either antigenic drift or antigenic shift reduces or eliminates the capacity of the local IgA antibody to neutralize a different strain of the virus.

Serum antibody

The level of serum antibody, primarily IgG, has been clearly shown to correlate with protection against influenza virus infection. This is only true if there is a close match between the existing antibody and the infecting strain of the virus.

IgG levels correlate with protection against influenza virus infection

In 80% of naturally acquired influenza virus infections, a systemic IgG antibody response can be demonstrated. With the virus essentially confined to the respiratory tract, it is unclear how systemic IgG reaches the target virus. It has already been stated that in the nasal secretions of humans infected with the Type A influenza virus, there is a preponderance of locally secreted IgA antibody. Also, the concentration of IgG antibody in the nasal wash has been reported to be 350 times less than that in the serum of infected individuals. However, it has been proposed that the observed protective efficacy of systemic anti-influenza IgG antibody is due to the relatively high levels of IgG antibody (compared with IgA) transudated from the circulation into the secretions that bathe the lower respiratory tract. This suggests that most cases of human influenza infection are actually initiated in the lower, rather than the upper, regions of the respiratory tract.

There is evidence that this may be the case. Nevertheless, a significant proportion of influenza infections are probably initiated either solely in the upper respiratory tract or may arise as a result of invasion of both the upper and lower reaches of the respiratory tract. This would therefore provide an explanation for the importance of local IgA antibody in protection against infection by these viruses (Table 3.1).

Protection and clearance

Protection against influenza virus infection is primarily effected through humoral immune mechanisms. The importance of cell-mediated immunity in the early stages of infection is minimal. As already mentioned, the major role of cellular immune mechanisms is in limiting the spread of an already established infection, and clearance of the virus from the body through the destruction of infected cells. These activities lead to elimination of the virus from the host and termination of the infection.

Influenza virus infections are eliminated in the host through the action of the cell-mediated immune system

Further reading

Anderson PJ. Factors promoting pathogenicity of influenza virus. *Semin Respir Infect* 1991; **6**: 3–10

Bender BS, Small PA. Influenza: pathogenesis and host defense. *Semin Respir Infect* 1992; **7**: 38–45

Seo SH, Webster RG. Tumor necrosis factor alpha exerts powerful anti-influenza virus effects in lung epithelial cells. *J Virol* 2002; **76**: 1071–6

4. Clinical assessment

Symptoms in adults
Symptoms in children
Influenza virus pneumonia
Diagnosis
Influenza in pregnancy
Management overview

Infection by the Type A and B influenza viruses usually occurs in winter, with most outbreaks in the UK occurring during December–March. The incidence of 'influenza-like illness' (episodes where the patient is showing typical symptoms of influenza without confirmation by laboratory diagnosis) reported by general practitioners in the UK varies annually, but cases are seen in most years. In the UK, a weekly incidence of influenza-like illnesses greater than 400 per 100 000 of the population is considered to constitute an infection rate of epidemic proportions.

Symptoms in adults

Influenza caused by either the Type A or B viruses is an acute infection with an incubation period of two or three days, and is a distinct clinical entity. Typically, the uncomplicated infection in adults is a tracheobronchitis with the additional involvement of the small airways. In addition to a high temperature (38–40 °C), the patient normally suffers an abrupt onset of malaise, headache, chills and myalgia in the limbs and back, and will be confined to bed for a few days. A dry nonproductive cough, occasionally accompanied by pharyngitis and nasal obstruction, may arise as the infection progresses.

Uncomplicated influenza in a healthy individual lasts from three to seven days. The fever starts to decline approximately three days after onset of the symptoms. The patient's temperature is usually back to normal five or six days after the onset. Although the physical findings are generally minimal, the patient can appear quite toxic and a generalized weakness may persist in some individuals for a week or so after recovery from the major clinical signs and symptoms. Many patients with genuine influenza virus infection are so ill that they will voluntarily take to their beds and are reluctant to exert themselves. Influenza infection is normally more severe in cigarette smokers.

Although most influenza infections during an epidemic are clinically typical of influenza, a minority are either asymptomatic or manifest as simple rhinitis, sometimes accompanied by pharyngitis. The symptoms of uncomplicated influenza in adults and their duration are shown in Figure 4.1.

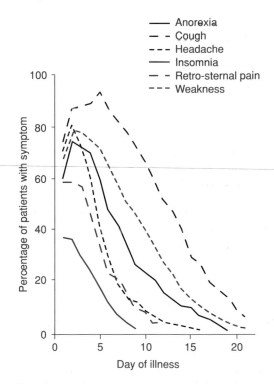

Figure 4.1
Frequency and duration of symptoms in 148 patients infected with the Type A/Hong Kong/68 influenza virus. From Hobson *et al.* 1972.

Symptoms in children

In children and younger individuals, influenza is generally of shorter duration, although the symptoms are essentially the same as in adults. There is a higher incidence of asymptomatic and minor infections in preschool and young schoolchildren than in adults. This is a factor associated with spread of the viruses by these cohorts of the population. Nevertheless, children can develop severe influenza infections, with high fever and occasionally febrile convulsions.

Symptoms that are seen more frequently in children than adults include:

- infections associated with the lower respiratory tract, such as croup and pneumonia
- extrapulmonary manifestations, such as vomiting, abdominal pain and myositis.

Myositis

Myositis is more commonly associated with Type B rather than Type A influenza virus infection, and usually presents as the child is recovering from the illness. The first symptoms are acute pain and tenderness, particularly in the gastrocnemius and soleus muscles, resulting in extremely painful walking. Serum creatine phosphokinase levels are usually transiently elevated. Occasionally, myositis occurs as a result of direct viral invasion of the muscle and the clinical symptoms are synchronous with the other, more usual, manifestations of influenza. Most patients recover completely after three to four days, although myoglobinuria and renal failure can sometimes occur. Very rarely, cardiac myositis occurs with classic ECG changes of myositis, sometimes accompanied by tachydysrhythmias. The cardiac enzymes may be greatly elevated.

> The symptoms of influenza are essentially the same in children and adults, but last longer in adults

Reye's syndrome

Reye's syndrome is very occasionally associated with influenza virus infection in children, particularly during or following long-term aspirin therapy. The symptoms are consistent with acute encephalopathy with cerebral oedema. The patient usually has raised cerebrospinal fluid (CSF) pressure but normal CSF microscopy and biochemistry. This condition is associated with fatty degeneration of the liver manifest as abnormal liver function tests and occasionally jaundice. However, this rare disease may be associated with other non-influenzal trigger factors.

Influenza virus pneumonia

Complications involving the lower respiratory tract can occur following influenza virus infection in both adults and children. These are usually seen in the groups particularly at risk from the infection, such as the elderly, in whom 80–90% of all influenza-related deaths occur. Individuals with chronic obstructive airways disease or other cardiopulmonary diseases are also at particular risk. Nevertheless, in the 1957 Asian influenza pandemic, when primary influenza virus pneumonia was first clearly documented, it was reported that one-quarter of these primary pneumonia cases occurred in normal, healthy individuals.

> Symptoms of influenza virus pneumonia include a rapid respiration rate, tachycardia, cyanosis, high fever and hypotension

Clinically, following the onset of influenza, a viral pneumonia accompanied by an overwhelming toxaemia characteristically develops within 24 hours. The symptoms include a rapid respiration rate, tachycardia, cyanosis, high fever and hypotension. Hypoxaemia and death may follow between one and four days later. Such severe and fatal infections are usually associated with the Type A influenza viruses, but the pathogenesis of these toxaemic symptoms is not well understood.

The virus replicates in and is confined to the epithelial cells of the respiratory tract. It is rarely detected in the blood of infected individuals. Under *in vitro* conditions, however, the virus can enter leukocytes, lymphocytes and macrophages, and exert certain biological effects on them.

A chest X-ray of a patient with influenza virus pneumonia usually shows patchy consolidation in two or more lobes (Figure 4.2). Cavitation or pleural effusion implies bacterial superinfection. The pneumonia is an interstitial pneumonitis with severe hyperaemia and broadening of the alveolar walls together with a mononuclear cell infiltration accompanied by capillary dilatation and thrombosis. This pathological presentation is also produced by other viruses infecting the lower respiratory tract.

In influenza virus pneumonia, the virus replicates in the alveolar epithelial cells. Influenza-specific antigen can be detected in these cells and in alveolar macrophages. Initial improvement in those destined to survive occurs five to 16 days after onset of the pneumonia. In general there

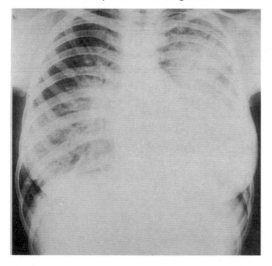

Figure 4.2
A typical X-ray presentation of fatal influenza virus pneumonia in an adult patient, showing acute lung congestion spread diffusely from the hilar region into the periphery and irregular soft mottling. [Reproduced from Mulder J, Hers JF. *Influenza*. Wolters Noordhoff, 1972.]

are no lasting problems, although a minority of patients develop a diffuse interstitial fibrosis accompanied by impaired lung function.

> During the major pandemic of 1957, a quarter of primary influenza virus pneumonia cases occurred in otherwise apparently healthy individuals

Diagnosis

Differential diagnosis of influenza is usually not possible on clinical grounds in non-epidemic periods, as the respiratory tract manifestations of the infection are common to those produced by other respiratory tract pathogens. During an influenza epidemic, however, the disease is reasonably easy to diagnose clinically and without laboratory help. Moreover, during an epidemic attributable to influenza Types A or B, an adult with a diffuse interstitial pneumonia is likely to be suffering from influenza virus pneumonia.

A complete and reliable diagnosis of the infection can only be established with laboratory help:

- by recovery of the virus from clinical samples such as throat or nasal swabs or washings by culture
- by the detection of specific viral proteins or viral genetic material in such clinical specimens
- by the demonstration of increasing specific anti-influenza antibodies in serum or nasal washes.

Influenza in pregnancy

During the two or three years following the appearance of a novel pandemic influenza virus strain, there is an increased risk of women developing fatal influenzal disease during the second or third trimester of pregnancy. This increased risk was reported after both the 1918 and the 1957 Type A influenza virus pandemics.

There is no definitive association of influenza virus infection with either congenital anomalies or haematological malignancies. The virus has only very rarely been isolated from either the maternal bloodstream or the fetus.

> After a novel virus pandemic, pregnant women are at risk of developing fatal influenzal disease

Management overview

The management of influenza is based on the annual vaccination of those populations considered to be at the greatest risk of infection from either the viruses or sequelae, such as secondary bacterial infections. Such groups include:

- those aged 65 years and above
- other groups who are immunocompromised for whatever reason

- those with chronic respiratory or heart disease
- diabetics.

See Chapter 6 (p 29) for more detail on the use of influenza virus vaccines in the management of infection. Information on the ever-increasing numbers and use of anti-influenza drugs is given in Chapter 7 (p 39).

Further reading

Hobson D, Beare AS, Ward-Gardner A. Haemagglutination-inhibiting serum antibody titres as an index of the response of volunteers to intranasal infection with live attenuated strains of influenza virus. *Proc Symp on Live Influenza Vaccines* Zagreb: Yugoslav Academy of Sciences and Arts, 1972: 73–84.

Murphy BR, Webster RG. Orthomyxoviruses. In: Fields BN, Knipe DM, Chanock RM *et al.* (eds) *Fields' Virology* (*Volume 1*) 2nd. Philadelphia, PA: Raven Press, 1990; 1091–152.

Oliviera EC, Marik PE, Colice G. Influenza pneumonia: a descriptive study. *Chest* 2001; **119**: 1717.

5. Complications and 'at risk' populations

The immunocompromised patient
Secondary bacterial complications
Conclusions

Severe and frequently fatal complications are caused by secondary bacterial infections in certain 'at risk' groups of the population. These groups include:

- the elderly or debilitated, particularly those aged 75 years and above
- persons with chronic respiratory disease, including asthmatics and chronic bronchitics
- diabetics
- individuals with chronic and ischaemic heart disease
- immunocompromised individuals
- individuals with renal disease
- residents of closed institutions, where attack rates during an influenza epidemic may be extremely high.

If associated with Type A influenza viruses, secondary bacterial infections can be particularly harmful

---

In persons over 65 years with two or more high-risk conditions for influenza, the death rate attributable to influenza is 0.8% compared to 0.02% in those aged 45–64 with no chronic disease conditions. In the over 65 age group, people at the highest risk of catching influenza are those who have cardiovascular disease in combination with either chronic obstructive pulmonary disease (COPD) or diabetes mellitus.

The immunocompromised patient

All individuals in the 'at risk' groups of the population will be compromised to some degree with respect to one or more elements of their nonspecific, or specific, immune defences. This situation may arise through:

- the natural course of events (for example, there is a decline in the immune response with advancing years, due to the involution of the thymus gland: this is a process that results in a reduction in the functioning mass of the gland, producing a T-cell insufficiency)
- a decrease in T-lymphocyte function in the elderly, resulting in a drop in both the quality and quantity of the T-cell help delivered to other components of the immune system, including B-cells.

These factors, together with the elimination of lymphocytes of various specificities throughout adult life, result in a characteristically changed immunological repertoire in the elderly. In some people, an immunocompromised state or an inadequately functioning respiratory tract may have been acquired through occupational disease or excessive smoking.

The number of young people at risk of death during an influenza virus epidemic or pandemic has increased due to the increased survival rates of:

- children with congenital diseases, eg cystic fibrosis and inherited immunodeficiencies
- organ transplant patients
- HIV patients.

Secondary bacterial complications

Each year many thousands of deaths are attributable to secondary bacterial diseases following an influenza virus infection. The bacteria most frequently involved are *Streptococcus pneumoniae*, *Staphylococcus aureus* and *Haemophilus influenzae*. Infection with *S. aureus* affects the lung by causing oedema, hyperaemia, haemorrhaging, consolidation and formation of pus (see Figure 5.1).

Pathogenesis

Interestingly, although influenza viruses preferentially replicate in the epithelial cells of the upper respiratory tract, they can also grow in leukocytes and peripheral blood monocytes. The viruses are able – at least under laboratory conditions – to induce apoptosis (programmed cell death) in these cells through the activity of the nonstructural protein NS1. Infection of humans with influenza Type A viruses has been reported to cause a severe but transient leukopenia. In recent experimental infections, some volunteers (around 10%) developed a severe T-cell lymphopenia and a moderate B-cell lymphopenia. However, 90% of the volunteers did show normal serum antibody responses. During the inflammatory processes associated with both uncomplicated influenza virus infection and secondary bacterial infections, leukocytes are recruited into the airways. Apoptosis of these cells is triggered by the infecting virus and could play a role in pathogenesis. This programmed cell death allows increased bacterial growth and multiplication because the efficiency of a major bacterial defence mechanism, the uptake and destruction of bacteria by leukocytes, is reduced.

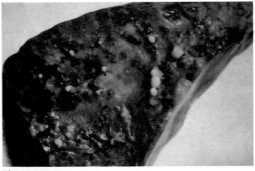

Figure 5.1
Gross appearance at post mortem of lung following *Staphylococcus aureus* infection secondary to influenza virus infection, showing oedema, hyperaemia, haemorrhaging, consolidation and the presence of pus.
[Reproduced from Mulder J, Hers JF. *Influenza*. Wolters Noordhoff, 1972.]

Morbidity

In the UK, deaths from secondary bacterial infection subsequent to an influenza virus infection are reflected in the figures of excess mortality, derived from the annually published national mortality statistics. The figures of excess mortality represent the number of deaths actually observed above that of the expected deaths over a given time period. In a winter period showing epidemic activity of a Type A influenza virus, the excess mortality figures are considerably higher than in a non-epidemic winter. This is almost entirely due to deaths (mainly in the elderly) from secondary bacterial pneumonias following influenza virus infection. Table 5.1 shows the excess deaths in England and Wales for all age groups of the population over 10 winters spanning the time period from 1989/90 through to 1998/99. The table indicates that most deaths were seen in the winters of 1989/90 and 1996/97.

Over the winter of 1994/95 there were fewer observed deaths than were expected, although this was a period of prolonged Type B influenza activity (Table 5.1). This indicates the lower virulence of this virus compared with the Type A viruses. Furthermore, the H3N2 subtype of the Type A virus was active during all but three of these winters, with Type B influenza being the active virus in 1990/91 and 1992/93 as well as in 1994/95. There was no significant outbreak associated with the H1N1 Type A influenza subtype over this period, suggesting either a greater degree of immunity to this virus in the general population, or a lower intrinsic H1N1 virus virulence, or a combination of both factors.

Annual data on the excess number of people presenting with influenza-like illness (over the baseline rate of incidence) are issued from the Royal College of General Practitioners (RCGP). These excess numbers of consultations, for all age groups of the population, are also shown in Table 5.1. During 1989–1999, an average of 421 872 individuals per year sought consultations for influenza-like illnesses.

Table 5.1
Excess deaths and estimates of excess consultations for influenza-like illness in England and Wales over 10 influenza seasons

Influenza season	Influenza virus type/subtype active	Duration of epidemic (weeks)	Excess deaths in all age groups	Excess consultations for influenza-like illness in all age groups
1989/90	H3N2	10	25 202	831 621
1990/91	B	12	11 356	276 064
1991/92	H3N2	11	6 707	266 525
1992/93	B	9	4 358	213 820
1993/94	H3N2	10	16 455	578 427
1994/95	B	14	−1 562	357 460
1995/96	H3N2	11	15 199	430 887
1996/97	H3N2	13	27 587	782 190
1997/98	H3N2	9	4 873	130 858
1998/99	H3N2	9	15 369	350 872
Mean	–	–	12 554	421 872

[Adapted from: Goddard NL, Joseph CA, Zambon M *et al*. Influenza surveillance in England and Wales: October 1999 to May 2000. *Commun Dis Public Health* 2000; **3**: 261–6. With kind permission of the PHLS Communicable Disease Surveillance Centre ©PHLS.]

Clinical features

There are certain conditions that act as significant risk factors when sufferers contract influenza. Gradually scientists are beginning to understand the underlying factors that may precipitate serious or even fatal illness in these individuals. The common theme is the immunocompromised state, but this has many differing facets, which may be manifest in a variety of ways.

Chronic obstructive pulmonary disease (COPD)

In COPD, excessive smoking, environmental pollution and prior infections may cause inflammatory damage to conducting airways and impair mucociliary clearance. This can lead to bacterial superinfection of the respiratory tract by, eg *Haemophilus influenzae*, *Moraxella catarrhalis* and *Streptococcus pneumoniae*. Indeed, the patient is often colonized by these bacteria. Exacerbations associated with COPD include shortness of breath, cough and sputum production. Infection by influenza Type A and B viruses can lead to serious lower respiratory tract episodes involving one or more of the species mentioned above.

Bronchiectasis

Bronchiectasis is a chronic condition of the respiratory tract. In bronchiectasis, as in COPD, the bronchial tree is heavily colonized by bacteria and the patient suffers a chronic cough, haemoptysis, copious sputum production and general ill health. The disease is usually the result of a severe bacterial respiratory tract infection, such as whooping cough or pulmonary tuberculosis. It presents as an irreversible and abnormal dilatation of the bronchi with chronic inflammatory and fibrotic changes.

Cystic fibrosis

Cystic fibrosis is a genetically inherited autosomal recessive disease. In cystic fibrosis, the respiratory tract of affected neonates, infants and children is colonized by bacteria such as *Staphylococcus aureus* and *Haemophilus influenzae*. In patients with advanced disease, various species of mucoid and nonmucoid pseudomonads also cause colonization. The viscous respiratory tract secretions in patients with cystic fibrosis tend to block the small airways, producing bronchiectasis.

Patients with a compromised respiratory tract who contract influenza have an increased risk of severe or fatal bacterial overgrowth and invasion of the lungs

Ischaemic heart disease

The deaths occurring in individuals with ischaemic heart disease during an influenza epidemic may be explained by:

- the increased myocardial demands associated with the fever and hypoxia caused by viral infection
- the viral myocarditis that can sometimes occur in influenza virus infection.

In addition, the inflammatory response accompanying the infection may create a prothrombotic state, leading to an acute thrombotic cardiovascular event.

HIV

HIV infection impairs cellular immune responses, humoral immunity is also affected. Resistance to infection by the influenza virus is primarily achieved through the presence of antibodies to the viral surface proteins at the time of infection. Recovery from the disease is mediated partly by cellular immune mechanisms – principally through the action of cytotoxic T-lymphocytes. Thus, individuals with HIV infection or with acquired immunodeficiency syndrome (AIDS) will be at particular risk during an influenza epidemic.

Diabetes

Individuals over 65 years of age with diabetes mellitus who contract influenza have a six-fold increased risk of hospitalization, and the mortality in such hospitalized persons is substantially increased. The risk from influenza virus infection in this group appears to be related to the cardiovascular complications of diabetes mellitus rather than to the diabetes itself. Infection with the influenza virus, or the complications associated with the infection may, however, cause a loss of

metabolic control in diabetic patients. This results in an increase in glycosylated serum proteins and in ketoacidosis. Therefore, the hospitalization rate increases, as does the incidence of long-term complications and the mortality rate.

Asthma

In children suffering from asthma, influenza virus infection leads to exacerbations of wheezing and increased risk of hospitalization. It has been estimated that 24–85% of all asthma attacks in children are associated with viral respiratory tract infections – respiratory syncytial virus (RSV) infection is the most common, but influenza can also aggravate asthma.

Smoking

Smoking has not been reported to be a significant risk factor for hospitalizations or fatalities despite the fact that smoking has been reported to be a risk factor for contracting influenza virus infection both in healthy young men and in a general population with a mean age of 44 years. However, infections are said to be more severe in cigarette smokers. Smoking does not appear to be a special risk factor for the elderly.

Smoking has been reported as a risk factor for contracting influenza virus infection, but not for hospitalizations or fatalities

Conclusions

Influenza continues to have a considerable impact on the health of the nation. There is a potentially severe or fatal outcome in the significant and increasing proportion of the population that is already at some degree of risk due to age and/or chronic ill health. This is so, despite the availability since the 1970s of a vaccine known to be both safe and, at least where there is concordance between the infecting virus and the viral antigens present in the vaccine, effective. The problem of influenza thus resides in the peculiar properties of the virus itself. It remains a continuing challenge to find a novel vaccine or means of immunization, or to discover a novel drug that can successfully overcome – or at the very least markedly diminish – the frequent and regular effects of this virus on human communities around the world.

Further reading

Couch RB. Influenza: prospects for control. *Ann Intern Med* 2000; **133**: 992–8.

Cruijff M, Thijs C, Govaert T *et al.* The effect of smoking on infuenza, influenza vaccination efficacy and on the antibody response to influenza vaccination. *Vaccine* 1999; **17**: 426–32.

Das P. Flu experts feel countries are unprepared for a future pandemic. *Lancet* 2001; **357**; 1419.

Kramarz P, DeStefano F, Garguillo PM *et al.* Influenza vaccination in children with asthma in health maintenance organizations. Vaccine Safety Datalink Team. *Vaccine* 2000; **18**: 2288–94.

Nichols JE, Niles JA, Roberts NJ Jr. Human lymphocyte apoptosis after exposure to influenza A virus. *Virology* 2001; **73**: 5921–9.

Nicholson KG. Impact of influenza and respiratory syncytial virus on mortality in England and Wales from January 1975 to December 1990. *Epidemiol and Infect* 1996; **116**: 51–63.

Simonsen L, Clarke MJ, Schonberger LB *et al.* Pandemic versus epidemic influenza mortality: a pattern of changing age distribution. *J Infect Dis* 1998; **178**: 53–60.

Webster RG. Immunity to influenza in the elderly. *Vaccine* 2000; **18**: 1686–9

6. Immunization

Efficacy
Groups recommended for vaccination
Vaccine production
Safety
Problems
Determination of immunogenicity
Novel vaccines
Local and systemic immune
    mechanisms
Use of vaccines in general practice

The first vaccines against influenza, developed and used in the 1950s and 1960s, consisted simply of the complete virus particles killed by treatment with formaldehyde. They were relatively crude and impure and liable to give rise to both cutaneous reactions at the injection site and systemic side-effects, particularly fever, in an unacceptable proportion of the recipients. Although such vaccines, albeit in a much more highly purified form, remain available today, the influenza virus vaccines currently in use in the UK contain only the surface haemagglutinin (HA) and neuraminidase (NA) proteins of the virus (Figure 6.1). These nonliving protein preparations are thus extremely pure and are well tolerated by recipients following intramuscular injection. They are the only form of influenza virus vaccine recommended for children under 12 years of age, as killed whole-virus vaccines may elicit systemic reactions, including high fever, in this age group.

> Surface antigen vaccines are the only form of influenza virus vaccine recommended for children under 12 years of age

Efficacy

Although their record on safety in all age groups of the population is excellent, surface antigen influenza virus vaccines do not demonstrate the very highest degree of efficacy (both in terms of the humoral and cell-mediated immune responses they induce, and in the protection rates they achieve). This is especially true when there is a lack of close concordance between the viral antigens present in the vaccine and the viral strains circulating and causing infection in the general population. Even when close concordance does exist, there is often a lowered vaccine efficacy because of underlying problems relating to poor immune responses in recipients of the vaccine. These decreased immune responses may be due to:

- immune senescence in the elderly
- an immune system compromised through infections with viruses such as HIV, or treatments with immunosuppressive drugs received by cancer or organ transplant patients.

Patients in these groups are at increased risk of severe or even fatal illness during an influenza virus epidemic. Hence, these groups are among the primary targets for influenza vaccination. It is clear that improvements in the nature of the vaccine or in the mode of its administration to the patient are necessary in order to provide adequate protection through the regularly occurring influenza virus epidemics.

> Primary targets for influenza vaccination are patients with compromised immune systems

Groups recommended for vaccination

Table 6.1 lists those groups for whom influenza vaccination is currently recommended in the UK. In addition, it is recommended that immunization be offered to all healthcare workers involved in the delivery of patient care and support. It is particularly

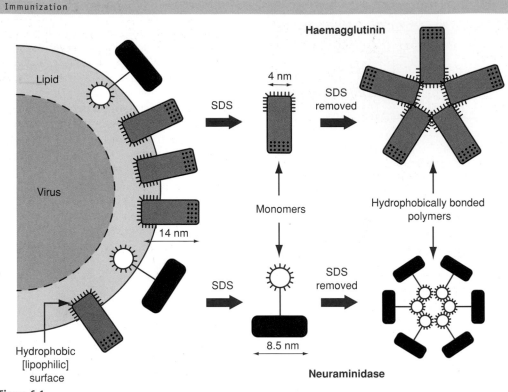

Figure 6.1
Schematic diagram showing the principles employed in the preparation of a surface antigen influenza vaccine, SDS = sodium dodecyl sulfate. [Adapted from Laver WG, Valentine RC. Morphology of the isolated haemagglutinin and neuraminidase subunits of influenza virus. *Virology* 1969; **38**: 105–19. With kind permission from Academic Press, Florida, USA]

important that these groups have some protection during an influenza epidemic, as the reduction in such support at these times may impose major strains on the capacity of the health services to deal with the epidemic. This can then lead to the development of an emergency situation.

Although vaccination is not recommended for healthy children and adults under the age of 65, infection in these groups may still lead to an economic burden in terms of the number of working days and schooldays lost during even a mild influenza outbreak.

> It is recommended that immunization be offered to all healthcare workers involved in the delivery of patient care and support

Vaccine production

Influenza virus vaccines are currently manufactured in embryonated hen's eggs. The H3N2, H1N1 and B influenza virus strains whose surface HA and NA proteins are to be incorporated in the vaccine for Europe are selected by the World Health Organization (WHO) in March each year. This selection is based on information obtained through the Influenza Surveillance Network, which involves over 100 laboratories around the world that report to four WHO collaborating centres. The Influenza Surveillance Network monitors and reports on the incidence and severity of influenza outbreaks worldwide. The Network particularly focuses on the strains of virus causing these epidemics, including any changes seen in the surface proteins. Any

Table 6.1
Groups recommended for annual vaccination against influenza

- All persons aged over 65 years
- Individuals of all ages with chronic respiratory disease:
  - chronic obstructive pulmonary disease
  - bronchiectasis
  - asthma
  - cystic fibrosis
- Individuals of all ages with chronic cardiac disease
- Individuals of all ages with chronic renal disease
- Individuals with diabetes mellitus
- Immunosuppressed individuals:
  - leukaemias and other cancers
  - organ transplant patients
  - HIV/AIDS patients
- Individuals in long-stay residential accommodation

Influenza virus vaccines are produced in a licensed cell system, which is usually well characterized, pathogen-free embryonated hen's eggs

detectable change in the antigenic nature of the surface proteins (particularly HA) of a newly isolated strain of influenza virus, which may indicate the possible development of a widespread outbreak or epidemic of influenza, will result in a recommendation to the vaccine manufacturers that these antigens be included in the vaccine for use in the following winter. The European manufacturers then have from April to October to prepare a sufficient amount of the recommended vaccine formulation.

Preparation of the vaccine commences with the propagation of the recommended virus strains in a licensed cell system – usually well characterized and pathogen-free embryonated hen's eggs. The licensed cell system is then inoculated with each of the current strains destined for use in the vaccine. This is done for the Type A influenza viruses with well categorized, laboratory adapted and genetically stable strains of influenza H3N2 and H1N1 that are of low or no virulence for humans, and are also capable of growing to very high levels in eggs.

These 'master' H3N2 and H1N1 strains will then undergo genetic reassortment with the current H3N2 and H1N1 strains injected with them. This enables production of viruses carrying the genes and bearing the surface proteins of each of the currently circulating influenza viruses required in the vaccine. However, these viruses will also possess genes derived from the respective master strains that code for their internal proteins. Such reassortants will:

- contain all the internal proteins of the master strain
- grow well in eggs
- be highly characterized and genetically stable with respect to all their internal proteins, even though they carry the surface HA and NA proteins of the current viruses.

Subsequent growth of these reassortants produces large quantities of virus bearing the required surface proteins. These are removed from the virus, normally through the use of surface-active agents, and purified for use in the vaccine.

Reassortment techniques are not used for influenza Type B virus vaccines. However, surface HA and NA proteins from the current circulating Type B virus are used in the vaccine following:

- cultivation of the virus in embryonated eggs
- removal of the surface proteins using surface-active agents
- purification of the proteins.

The difficulties associated with influenza vaccine technology include poor growth of current virus strains in eggs, and problems in obtaining the required reassorted virus at the reassortment stage. Both of these problems can prolong the time taken for vaccine production, delay the availability of vaccine for widespread use and also affect the quantities of vaccine that can readily be prepared. The safety factors inherent in these procedures (especially the elimination of any potential virulence factors associated with the internal proteins of the cirulating wild-type viruses) are important, although in the face of an impending influenza pandemic caused by a strain of virus that is new to humans, large quantities of an effective, rapidly available vaccine will be needed urgently.

In recent years, a number of the major pharmaceutical companines have been researching and developing novel influenza vaccines using cell culture systems as a substrate for propagation of the virus rather than the embryonated hen's egg. Although such culture systems have some advantages over eggs for influenza virus growth, eg permitting a more appropiate structure for the surface HA protein antigen of the virus, there are concerns that it may be harder to achieve rapid, large-scale production of influenza vaccine in these cell culture systems.

Safety

The current surface protein influenza virus vaccines are very safe. They consist of the two Type A virus HA and NA antigens together with the HA and NA antigens from a single Type B influenza virus. In several studies in healthy adults, at dosage levels four times that currently used, these vaccines have been found to induce systemic reactions (such as raised temperature) no more frequently than in individuals receiving a placebo preparation.

These surface protein influenza virus vaccines are also safe in children under two years of age. Furthermore, there is no evidence of raised temperatures or febrile convulsions in this age cohort. These side-effects have been reported for the killed whole-virus vaccines, but such preparations are not available for use in the UK.

Most studies have reported a low level, about 5%, of local reactions at the injection site following administration of the commercially available surface protein influenza virus vaccines. These reactions are mild and transient, lasting only 24–48 hours. Local or systemic allergic reactions to the highly purified surface protein influenza virus vaccines are very uncommon. Most of the reactions probably occur in people with egg allergies and are precipitated by the minute amounts of egg protein that is residual in the vaccine. The use of the current egg-grown vaccines is contraindicated in individuals with egg allergies.

Exceptionally rarely, immunization against influenza has also been associated with Guillain–Barré syndrome.

> Vaccination is contraindicated in individuals with egg allergies

Problems

The limitations in efficacy of the current influenza virus vaccines have been mentioned earlier and are mainly due to two factors.

First, it has not proved possible to predict correctly the exact antigenic nature of the strains of virus that will be circulating during a forthcoming influenza season. Despite considerable theoretical and experimental work aimed at defining the nature of the mutations that take place in the virus genome, and searching for trends in past mutations in the genes coding for the surface proteins through the construction of phylogenetic trees, it is still impossible to anticipate these changes with any degree of accuracy. Therefore, in any given influenza epidemic, there will be a less than perfect match between the vaccine antigens and the circulating virus strains.

Second, the prime target groups at whom the vaccine is aimed – the elderly and the chronically ill – are often less than fully competent in their immune responses. The protection rates achieved following vaccination of these groups may be much lower than those elicited by the same vaccine in a healthy population. Some studies have reported protection rates as low as 20% in the elderly following immunization with a vaccine that matched the circulating influenza virus strains. Healthy young adults receiving the same vaccine under similar circumstances had a protection rate of 70%.

Determination of vaccine immunogenicity

The immunogenicity of current commercially available and novel experimental influenza virus vaccines is primarily assessed by determination of the levels of antibodies to the surface proteins of the virus (particularly the HA antigen) circulating in the blood of vaccine recipients. The level of such serum antibody that can be equated with a 50% chance of protection against infection by an influenza virus has been determined. European guidelines for the registration of influenza virus vaccines recommend that new, experimental influenza

vaccines should elicit such protective levels of antibody in 75% of vaccine recipients.

Novel vaccines

Since the current commercially available influenza vaccines do not always provide a high level of protection, there is considerable interest in the further improvement of these vaccines either:

- through modification of the vaccines themselves, or
- through the way in which they are delivered.

Natural infection by the influenza viruses is acquired via the respiratory tract, with the virus initiating its replication in the lining mucosal epithelial cells. Both the virological and the host defence factors (specific and nonspecific) associated with the initiation and progress of the infection are presented in Table 6.2.

It is unlikely that an influenza vaccine given by injection into the deltoid muscle of the upper arm will induce appropriate antibody levels in the secretions bathing either the upper or the

Table 6.2
Events associated with establishment of influenza virus infection in the respiratory tract

Viral event	Nonspecific host defence effector mechanisms operating	Specific immune host defence mechanisms that will operate if present
Initial presence at mucosal surface	Mucus viscosity Mucociliary escalator Protease enzymes present in local secretions	Nil
Attachment and entry into susceptible cells	Mucus viscosity Mucociliary escalator Protease enzymes in secretions	Locally produced IgA IgG transudated from the circulation
Replication inside susceptible cells	Interferon Apoptosis (programmed cell death)?	Nil
Presence and release of virus from infected cell surface	Natural killer cells	Cytotoxic T-lymphocytes Locally produced IgA IgG transudated from the circulation
Extracellular spread of virus in the respiratory tract	Complement	Locally produced IgA IgG transudated from the circulation

lower respiratory tract in the days and weeks following immunization. It is also unlikely that such antibody levels will be sustained over a whole influenza season. It is for these reasons that novel vaccines are under investigation.

Local and systemic immune mechanisms

The major antibody isotype present in mucosal secretions throughout the body is IgA. This is produced locally at the mucosal surfaces and is relatively short lived. The longer lasting IgG antibody isotype, which is the major isotype produced in response to parenteral antigenic stimulation, forms only a minor component of respiratory tract secretions. It is believed to enter these secretions by transudation from the blood vessels underlying the respiratory mucosa. This transudation is greatest when there is some degree of inflammation in the respiratory tract. Inflammation can be brought about by, for example infection with bacteria or viruses, including influenza. Ideally, to prevent infection of the respiratory tract mucosa by an invading influenza virus, the presence and immediate secretion of locally produced IgA antibody is an important prerequisite. The presence of such antibody in the secretions bathing the respiratory mucosal surfaces at the time of infection can prevent attachment of the virus to susceptible cells. If supported by nonspecific host defences, such as natural killer cells and interferon destroying those cells that do become infected by the virus, IgA should provide protection against the establishment of infection and development of the clinical symptoms of influenza. The closeness of the match between the anti-HA IgA antibodies and the HA protein present on the surface of the invading virus is also important here.

Intramuscular injection of the current influenza vaccines can promote high levels of durable systemic IgG antibodies and also memory cells that are able to respond in the event of subsequent infection. However, there will be a delay before these effector mechanisms are translated to, and are operating at, the

respiratory mucosal surfaces. The immune actions of IgG antibodies and memory cells may not be transudated to the respiratory secretions until the inflammatory effects resulting from the infection are well under way and the virus is established in the respiratory tract tissues. Therefore, a major role for these specific defence mechanisms may be in limiting the spread of the virus and clearing an influenza virus infection that is already established in the respiratory tract.

Delivery by nasal route

Because of the relevance of local specific immune mechanisms, particularly the activity of secretory IgA, in the prevention of influenza virus infection at the respiratory tract mucosal surfaces, the administration of an influenza vaccine via the nasal route (probably by means of a spray mechanism) is currently receiving considerable attention. If delivery of a surface protein influenza vaccine by this route can achieve high levels of local IgA antibody in nasal secretions, and if these levels can be sustained over the entire influenza season (perhaps through periodic 'top-up' intranasal spray inoculations), then an important component of the specific defences required to prevent the initiation and establishment of infection by the virus will have been implemented. This is probably not a feature of the current intramuscularly injected vaccines.

> Direct vaccine delivery by a nasal spray could achieve high levels of IgA antibody in nasal secretions. This is an important specific immune defence to prevent the establishment of infection

Use of vaccines in general practice

Although repeated annual vaccination against influenza has been a controversial issue in the past, it now appears this strategy has an overall beneficial effect rather than a neutral one. Furthermore, there is no available evidence of any detrimental effect of annual vaccination on either the immune response levels achieved or the degree of protection afforded by the vaccine.

In addition, healthcare workers have reported that current vaccines can reduce the hospitalization and mortality rates of elderly individuals with complications of influenza by approximately 50%. Furthermore, a 1995 report in the *Lancet* by Karl Nicholson's group shows that repeated annual vaccination of the elderly is beneficial as it reduces mortality in this group by 75%. This compares with a reduction of only 9% among persons in this cohort who receive the influenza vaccine for the first time. More recent reports by Keitel in 1997 and Beyer in 1999 indicate that the immune responses achieved following repeated annual immunization against influenza is at least as effective as that seen following a single vaccination. However, most workers agree that in the population as a whole, the protection rates achieved in any given year by the surface protein influenza virus vaccines range from 60 to 80%.

> Repeated annual vaccination of the elderly can reduce mortality by up to 75%

A comprehensive meta-analysis, completed in 1995 by Gross *et al* looked at 20 cohort observational studies in over 5000 elderly persons ranging in age from 65 to 101 years over a time period from 1968 to 1989. The study included three case-control studies, two cost-effectiveness studies and one randomized, double-blind, placebo-controlled study. Gross *et al* reported that vaccination of the elderly with conventional, inactivated influenza vaccine reduced the risks of pneumonia, hospitalization and death from infection by the influenza virus. Specifically, the pooled estimates of influenza vaccine efficacy indicated that vaccination of the elderly reduced:

- death rate by 68%
- hospitalization by 50%
- pneumonia by 53%
- repiratory illness by 56%

The authors concluded that influenza immunization is an indispensable part of the care of people aged 65 years or above and all physicians and public health organizations should be made aware of this.

A more recent meta-analysis of clinical trials by Beyer and colleagues, completed in 2001, compared certain experimental, live attenuated influenza virus vaccines against conventional inactivated influenza virus vaccines in over 2000 people of all ages. From the five studies in this meta-analysis it was found that efficacy, as determined by laboratory-confirmed diagnosis of influenza virus infection following either experimental challenge with wild-type influenza virus or by natural challenge during an epidemic of influenza, ranged from 68 to 100% with a mean of 78.2%. in four of these five studies there was either an identical or very close match between the influenza antigens present in the vaccine and those carried by the virus used for the experimental challenge, or by the virus naturally in circulation in the comminity (Figure 6.2).

The recommendation for annual administration of influenza virus vaccine is a burden for the community-residing vaccine recipient and the individual in a long-term residential care home, in terms of having an injection and making a visit to the GP. In addition, the annual vaccination programme against influenza in the UK creates an extremely heavy workload for the community and district nursing staff. At this time of year, their workload may already be increased for other reasons. Nurses have to visit patients unable to get to health centres and vaccinate residents in long-term accommodation homes.

Immunization rates

Across the UK, GP policies and rates for immunization against influenza vary widely. In a 1998 survey of influenza virus vaccination in primary care in central southern England, when national guidelines only advised immunization for individuals with specified high-risk medical conditions or for those residing in long-stay care facilities, only 11.5% overall and 64% of those >75 years of age had been immunized

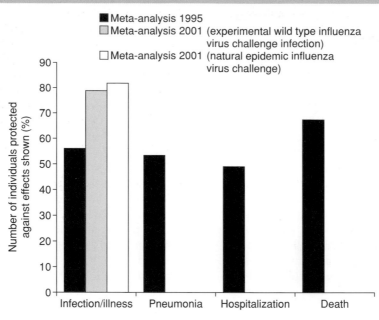

Figure 6.2
The percentages of individuals protected against infection or illness, pneumonia, hospitalization or death following immunization with conventional inactivated influenza vaccines as reported in two meta-analyses by Gross *et al* and Beyer *et al*.

against influenza. Currently available commercial influenza virus vaccines have not been popular with physicians in the UK. In a survey of 477 geriatricians in 1990, only 3% reported offering influenza vaccine to all their continuing care patients; 81% never used the vaccine. Of the 385 consultants who did not offer the vaccine, it was regarded as unnecessary by 56%, ineffective by 33% and too expensive for blanket use by 12%.

At the present time, GPs are reimbursed for vaccinating individuals in the 'at risk' groups and can purchase influenza vaccine at a good discount. Nevertheless, a small-scale survey carried out over the 1999–2000 winter, covering 76 general practices within the Merton, Sutton and Wandsworth Health Authority, indicated an overall influenza vaccination rate of only 50% in those aged >75 years. The range within individual practices was 7–97%. The study indicated that those practices achieving high coverage rates undertook personalized patient invitation and had well-organized clinics.

From the year 2000, GPs have received payments for vaccinating individuals aged ≥65 years. This may well have improved the coverage of influenza vaccination in this group of the population. Indeed, preliminary data from the Merton, Sutton and Wandsworth Health Authority suggest that all the practices surveyed increased their influenza vaccine coverage the following year. The overall immunization rate for the winter of 2000/01 was 62%, thereby meeting the required government coverage target for that year of 60%.

General perception

The regular outbreaks and epidemics of influenza, coupled with the widespread non-scientific and adverse press coverage of these events, are major factors that have given rise to the belief in both the general public and those charged with delivery of the vaccine that immunization against influenza has very little effect on the course of the disease. Of course at the population level, and as an epidemic takes hold and progresses, it is very easy to deride the effects of vaccination. However, despite the ongoing changes in the influenza viruses on an almost yearly basis, the predictions of which strains to include in the vaccine for any given year are becoming increasingly more accurate. In the current interpandemic state, where there has been no major antigenic change in the Type A influenza viruses for many years, vaccination is:

- saving lives
- reducing hospital admissions
- modifying the severity and duration of illness
- providing full protection against infection at the level of the individual.

Such information is derived from the annual data on the incidence of influenza in vaccinated and unvaccinated individuals gathered from well-conducted clinical trials and epidemiological studies.

However, this trend has not yet totally dispelled the concept that vaccination against influenza is a waste of time and money. This is partly because of the current inability to distinguish between true influenza virus infection and the 'influenza-like illnesses'. Influenza-like illnesses are primarily caused by respiratory syncytial virus (RSV), parainfluenza viruses and *Mycoplasma pneumoniae*.

One comment often received by GPs from people who are to be given the influenza injection is "I had the 'flu jab two years ago and I still had 'flu twice that winter". This can be countered with statements to the effect that besides influenza, there are a number of viruses and bacteria circulating in the community during winter that can cause very bad colds resembling 'flu (the 'influenza-like illnesses'), but these are not normally quite as severe as influenza nor are they normally life-threatening. Influenza can be very serious, and the influenza vaccine only protects against influenza not against these other winter respiratory tract illnesses.

Another question the physician may often be confronted with is "Will the 'flu jab make me ill?" The response is that it will not, as it is both a safe and a noninfectious preparation. In very few recipients of the vaccine there may be a soreness at the site of injection that lasts a few hours; in even fewer recipients there may be a slight fever and headache, but these should last no more than 24 hours. It is now also clear that the GP can safely say that the vaccine is now known to have a beneficial effect in preventing or ameliorating illness in people in the 'at risk' groups.

Further reading

Ahmed AH, Nicholson KG. The efficacy of influenza vaccine. *Reviews in Medical Microbiology* 1996; **7**: 23–30.

Ahmed AE, Nicholson KG, Nguyen-Van Tam JS. Reduction in mortality associated with influenza vaccine during the 1989–90 epidemic. *Lancet* 1995; **346**: 591–5.

Beyer WE, De Bruijn IA, Palache AM *et al*. Protection against influenza after annually repeated vaccination: a meta-analysis of serologic and field studies. *Arch Intern Med*. 1999 25; **159**: 182–8.

Beyer WE, Palache AM, de Jong JC, Osterhaus AD. Cold-adapted live influenza vaccine versus inactivated vaccine: systemic vaccine reactions, local and systemic antibody responses and vaccine efficacy. A meta-analysis. *Vaccine* 2002; **20**: 1340–53.

Brydak LB, Machala M. Humoral immune response to influenza vaccination in patients from high-risk groups. *Drugs* 2000; **60**: 35–53.

Carman WF, Elder AG, Wallace LA, McAulay K *et al*. Effects of influenza vaccination of health-care workers on mortality of elderly people in long-term care: a randomized controlled trial. *Lancet* 2000; **355**: 93–7.

De Bruijn IA, Remarque EJ, Jol-van der Zijde CM *et al*. Quality and quantity of humoral immune response in healthy elderly and young subjects after annually repeated influenza vaccination. *J Infect Dis* 1999; **179**: 31–6.

Eyles JE, Williamson ED, Alpar HO. Intranasal administration of influenza vaccines. *Biodrugs* 2000; **13**: 35–59.

Govaert TM, Thijs CT, Sprenger MW *et al*. The efficacy of influenza vaccination in elderly individuals. A randomized double-blind placebo controlled trial. *JAMA* 1994; **272**: 1661–5.

Gross PA, Hermogenes AW, Sacks HS *et al*. The efficacy of influenza vaccine in elderly persons. A meta-analysis and review of the literature. *Ann Intern Med* 1995; **123**: 518–27.

Hall GH. Antiflu or antideath vaccination. *Lancet* 2001; **357**: 2141.

Halperin SA, Smith B, Mabrouk T *et al*. Safety and immunogenicity of a trivalent, inactivated, mammalian cell culture-driven influenza vaccine in healthy adults, seniors and children. *Vaccine* 2002; **20**: 1240–7.

Keitel WA, Cate TR, Crouch RB *et al*. Efficacy of repeated annual immunization with inactivated influenza virus vaccines over a five year period. *Vaccine*. 1997; **15**: 1114–22.

Laver WG, Valentine RC. Morphology of the isolated haemagglutinin and neuraminidase subunits of influenza virus. *Virology* 1969; **38**: 105–19.

Lavanchy D. The importance of global surveillance of influenza. *Vaccine* 1999; **17**: S24–5.

Liddle BJ, Jennings R. Influenza vaccination in old age. *Age Ageing* 2001; **30**: 385–9.

Nichol KL. Clinical effectiveness and cost effectiveness of influenza vaccination among healthy working adults. *Vaccine* 1999: **17**: S67–73.

Nichol KL, Margolis KL, Wuorenma J, von Sternberg T. The efficacy and cost effectiveness of vaccination against influenza among elderly persons living in the community. *N Engl J Med* 1994; **331**: 778–84.

Pau MG, Ophorst C, Koldijk MH *et al*. The human cell line PER. C6 provides a new manufacturing system for the production of influenza vaccines. *Vaccine*. 2001; **19**: 2716–21.

Snacken R. Control of influenza. Public health policies. *Vaccine* 1999; **17(Suppl 3)**: S61–3.

7. Antiviral drugs for treatment and prevention

Amantadine and rimantadine
Neuraminidase inhibitors
Prophylaxis

Several drugs are now available for treatment and prevention of infection by the influenza virus, and these are summarized in Table 7.1.

Amantadine and rimantadine

The older agents, amantadine and rimantadine, are related substances that act by blocking the ion channel function of the influenza virus M2 protein. This protein, although a minor surface constituent of the influenza virus particle, is essential for virus replication. When functioning as an ion channel, the protein facilitates the entry of H$^+$ ions into the virus particle. This triggers a structural change in the virus haemagglutinin (HA) protein and degrades the viral envelope and matrix protein. This permits release of the viral nucleocapsid for migration through the cell cytoplasm and into the nucleus to initiate the next step of the replication cycle of the virus.

Amantadine and rimantadine are active against influenza A, but not against influenza B. Both agents are effective for the treatment of Type A influenza virus infection if treatment is begun within 48 hours of the onset of illness. They can shorten the illness by approximately one day. Both drugs are given orally and can cause nausea and vomiting in a small percentage of individuals. Unfortunately, amantadine is associated with certain unpleasant central nervous system side-effects such as:

- anxiety
- depression
- insomnia
- hallucinations.

These side-effects are dose-related and will resolve with discontinuation of the drug. Antiviral resistance can develop rapidly during use of either drug, and the resistant virus can then be transmitted from the index case to others.

Although these drugs are effective, their use in clinical influenza treatment has been limited as a result of their side-effect profile. Therefore, they have not been deployed for the treatment of community acquired influenza, but they have been used extensively in chemoprophylaxis.

Amantadine and rimantadine are:

- both effective for treatment of Type A influenza virus infection if treatment is begun within 48 hours of the onset of illness
- not active against Type B infections
- effective prophylactic agents against influenza
- relatively cheap

Neuraminidase inhibitors

Recently, several neuraminidase inhibitors have been developed that have a potent anti-influenza activity *in vitro* and also have clinical efficacy. They are active against both Type A and Type B influenza viruses. The neuraminidase (NA) surface protein of the virus is essential for the de-aggregation and release of newly synthesized virions from infected cells. Inhibition of this enzyme interrupts propagation of the influenza virus within the human respiratory tract. Specifically, the NA inhibitors are neuraminic (sialic) acid analogues, mimicking the structure of *N*-acetyl neuraminic acid (NANA). This complex sugar molecule is a component of the membrane of cells susceptible to influenza virus infection. It is also probably incorporated into the lipid envelopes of the virus particles as they are

Table 7.1
Antiviral agents for influenza

Antiviral agent	Trade name	Manufacturer	Influenza spectrum	Route of administration	Daily dosage for adults		Most common side-effects
					Prevention	Treatment	
Amantadine	Symmetrel	Endo Pharmaceuticals (USA)	Type A	Oral	200 mg	200 mg	Gastrointestinal and central nervous system
	Lysovir	Alliance (UK)					
Rimantadine†	Flumadine	Forest Laboratories (USA)	Type A	Oral	200 mg	200 mg	Gastrointestinal
Zanamivir	Relenza	GlaxoSmithKline	Types A and B	Oral inhalation	10 mg	20 mg	None
Oseltamivir†	Tamiflu	Roche	Types A and B	Oral	75 mg	150 mg	Gastrointestinal

†Not available in the UK

released from the host cells. NANA is an important membrane structure in the final stages of influenza virus replication, and virus interaction with the NA inhibitors both diverts and blocks their reactivity with NANA.

Only two drugs have so far been developed to the level of entry into the formulary:

- Zanamivir is a modification of Neu5Ac2en, a dehydrated neuraminic acid derivative.
- Oseltamivir is a similar molecule except that it has a cyclohexene ring and replaces a polyglycerol moiety with lipophilic side-chains.

Zanamivir can only be administered by inhalation, whereas oseltamivir can be taken by mouth. Both drugs are active against both the influenza Type A and the influenza Type B viruses.

A third drug, RWJ-270201, a cyclopentane derivative with a guanidinyl group and lipophilic side-chains, is currently under development in Phase II clinical trials and will be manufactured by Johnson & Johnson.

> Zanamivir and oseltamivir are effective against Type A and Type B influenza viruses

Efficacy

Both zanamivir and oseltamivir have been shown to be effective in the treatment of experimental influenza Type A virus infection in human studies. Both have also been shown to have significant antiviral effects in experimental influenza B infection. These trials are generally conducted in individuals who are susceptible to influenza virus infection – as evidenced by low titres of antibodies to the influenza virus HA protein in the circulation.

Following intranasal inoculation with influenza virus, untreated controls suffer fever and nasopharyngeal and otological manifestations of influenza virus infection. Furthermore, proinflammatory cytokines can be measured in nasal fluids taken from these individuals. Both zanamivir and oseltamivir reduce the incidence of these symptoms when used as prophylaxis in such trials. Both drugs prevent the shedding of virus and also infection-related respiratory illness. When used in experimental treatment (ie the drug is administered after the onset of symptoms), both drugs reduce symptom scores and duration of illness.

Treatment of community acquired influenza

Some clinical trials have been published regarding the use of zanamivir and oseltamivir in treatment of patients with influenza in the community (Table 7.2).

The evidence yielded by these studies has recently been reviewed by the Cochrane Collaboration. Neuraminidase inhibitors have been shown to shorten the duration of symptoms by one day. Across all studies, the time gained in returning to normal activities is half a day for laboratory-confirmed cases of influenza. The beneficial effect appears to be confined to patients in whom there is fever, and who are treated within 30 hours of the onset of symptoms. Zanamivir has been shown to reduce the frequency of antibiotic prescriptions for lower respiratory tract complications by 40%, but has not reduced prescriptions for presumed upper respiratory tract complications such as sinusitis and otitis.

So far, the neuraminidase inhibitors have not been extensively investigated in patients who are at the highest risk of serious complications of influenza. Such patients include the elderly and those with serious cardiopulmonary illness, such as chronic obstructive pulmonary disease. Although oseltamivir can be given orally, zanamivir must be given via an inhaler device – it is possible that both older and very young patients may not be able to deliver the drug effectively by this method.

Both drugs appear relatively safe. Zanamivir has very few side-effects, but oseltamivir does cause

Table 7.2
Neuraminidase inhibitors in the treatment of community acquired influenza

Treatment	Patients (% with proven influenza)	Age range (mean)	Duration of illness	Reduction in days to alleviation of symptoms in patients with influenza (median)	Comments	Investigator
Inhaled zanamivir 10 mg bid for 5 days	417 (63%)	≥13 years (32 years)	≤48 h	1 (5 vs 4) 3 (7 vs 4 in febrile)	3 days reduction in patients treated ≤30 h	Hayden et al (1997)
Inhaled zanamivir 10 mg bid for 5 days	455 (71%)	≥12 years (37 years)	<30 h and >30 h	1.5 (6.5 vs 5.0) 2.0 (6.5 vs 4.5 in febrile)	Reduced complications and antibiotics (15% vs 38%) in patients with underlying conditions. No effect in patients with symptoms >30 h	MIST Study Group (1998)
Oseltamivir 75 mg or 150 mg bid for 5 days	629 (60%)	18–65 years	≤36 h	1.4 (4.3 vs 2.9 vs 2.9)	Reduced complications	Treanor et al (2000)
Oseltamivir 75 mg or 150 mg bid for 5 days	719 (66%)	18–65 years	≤36 h	1.2–1.5 days (4.9 vs 3.6 vs 3.4)	No difference between doses	Nicholson et al (2000)

a significant incidence of nausea. When used for the treatment of children, inhaled zanamivir significantly reduced the time to alleviation of illness (by approximately one day). It has also reduced the time required for return to normal activities. Nebulized zanamivir is available for the treatment of younger children and infants. A liquid formulation of oseltamivir is effective in children aged between one and 10 years, and it reduces the frequency of complications leading to antibiotic prescriptions.

> The neuraminidase inhibitors have not yet been extensively investigated in patients who are at the highest risk of serious complications of influenza

Prophylaxis

Antiviral agents are valuable alternatives to vaccines for augmenting protection amongst vulnerable individuals, particularly patients who are immunodeficient. They are also very useful in the prevention of influenza within households and in institutional settings such as long-term care facilities for the elderly. Protection against infection is particularly important for:

- unvaccinated high-risk persons (the elderly or those with cardiopulmonary disease)
- high-risk persons when the vaccine–epidemic virus match is poor
- vaccinated persons during the window period after vaccination (10–14 days)
- unvaccinated healthcare workers
- staff in long-term care facilities during an influenza epidemic.

Currently, only amantadine (and outside the UK rimantidine) is approved for prophylaxis, but the neuraminidase inhibitors have the added advantage of being active against influenza Type B. Studies conducted over many years have shown that amantadine and rimantadine are very effective as prophylactic agents for the control of influenza Type A virus infections in nursing care facilities. Development of

resistance in this circumstance has not been a particular problem. Amantadine and rimantadine are relatively cheap drugs, which makes them preferred agents in this indication.

Both oseltamivir and zanamivir have been shown to prevent influenza, and their use in chemoprophylaxis has been reviewed by the Cochrane Collaboration.

The influenza virus neuraminidase inhibitors, when compared to placebo, are 74% effective in preventing naturally occurring cases of clinically defined influenza (95% confidence interval [CI]=50–87%), and 60% effective in preventing cases of laboratory-confirmed influenza virus infection (95% CI=76–33%). Several placebo-controlled studies of zanamivir and oseltamivir have now been conducted (Table 7.3).

Neuraminidase inhibitors have been administered to close contacts of index cases within 48 hours of initial clinical infection. Outcome measurements have included the infection rate in individual contacts, or the proportion of households in which new cases have been proven using laboratory methods. Zanamivir and oseltamivir appear to be equally effective and are of similar cost (considerably higher than that of amantadine). However, ease of administration favours the use of oseltamivir in the context of long-term care facilities. Administration of zanamivir requires good hand–eye coordination, lung function and comprehension. In the future, if neuraminidase inhibitors become licensed for this indication, they would probably be administered for 7–14 days in prophylactic situations.

With the increased understanding of the events that are involved in the growth and replication of influenza viruses at the molecular and cellular level, and the increased awareness of the interactions of the virus with a variety of host cell defence mechanisms, there is hope that the rate of discovery of new anti-influenza drugs will both continue and amplify.

Table 7.3
Neuraminidase inhibitors in chemoprophylaxis

Drug	No. of subjects	Exposure	Intervention	Outcome measurement	Result	Comment	Investigator
Zanamivir (Zm)	575	Close community contacts	Intranasal Zm (10 mg), inhaled Zm, or both in intranasal and inhaled Zm or placebo for 5 days	Rate of influenza contacts	Inhaled Zm reduced influenza rate	Intranasal Zm was ineffective	Kaiser et al (2000)
Zanamivir (Zm)	837	Family or household contacts	Inhaled Zm (10 mg) to household contacts of influenza cases or placebo for 5 days	Proportion of households with a secondary case	Zm reduced households with secondary cases: 19% (placebo) versus 4% Zm	No Zm resistance emerged	Hayden et al (2000)
Oseltamivir (Os)	955	Family or household contacts	Oseltamivir orally (75 mg) or placebo for 7 days	Rate of secondary clinical influenza in individuals and households	Os significantly reduced secondary cases and rates of secondary household infections. Viral shedding also reduced in contacts	Os side-effects similar to placebo	Welliver et al (2001)
Oseltamivir (Os)	236	Nursing home residents during natural influenza B index residential epidemic	Oseltamivir (75 mg) orally for 7 days	Secondary case rate compared to historical control without oseltamivir	Secondary case rate reduced from 19% to 10%	No placebo	Parker et al (2001)

Further reading

Anonymous. Randomised trial of efficacy and safety of inhaled zanamivir in treatment of influenza A and B virus infections. The MIST (Management of Influenza in the Southern Hemisphere Trialists) Study Group. *Lancet* 1998; **352**: 1877–81.

Gubareva LV, Kaiser L, Hayden FG. Influenza virus neuraminidase inhibitors. *Lancet* 2000; **355**: 827–35.

Hayden FG. Amantadine and rimantadine – clinical aspects. In: Richman DD (ed.) *Antiviral Drug Resistance*. Chichester, Wiley: 1996: 59–71.

Hayden FG, Osterhaus AD, Treanor JJ *et al*. Efficacy and safety of the neuraminidase inhibitor zanamivir in the treatment of influenzavirus infections. GG167 Influenza Study Group. *N Engl J Med* 1997; **337**: 874–80.

Hayden FG, Gubareva LV, Monto AS, *et al*. Inhaled zanamivir for the prevention of influenza in families. Zanamivir Family Study Group. *N Engl J Med* 2000; **343**: 1282–9.

Jefferson T, Demicheli V, Deeks J, Rivetti D. Neuraminidase inhibitors for preventing and treating influenza in healthy adults (Cochrane Review). In: *The Cochrane Library*, issue 1. Oxford: Update Software, 2002.

Kaiser L, Henry D, Flack NP *et al*. Short-term treatment with zanamivir to prevent influenza: results of a placebo-controlled study. *Clin Infect Dis* 2000; **30**: 587–9.

Nicholson KG, Aoki FY, Osterhaus AD *et al*. Efficacy and safety of oseltamivir in treatment of acute influenza: a randomized controlled trial. Neuraminidase Inhibitor Flu Treatment Investigator Group. *Lancet* 2000; **355**: 1845–50.

Parker R, Loewen N, Skowronski D. Experience with oseltamivir in the control of a nursing home influenza B outbreak. *Can Commun Dis Rep* 2001; **27**: 37–40.

Treanor JJ, Hayden FG, Vrooman PS *et al*. Efficacy and safety of the oral neuraminidase inhibitor oseltamivir in treating acute influenza: a randomized controlled trial. US Oral Neuraminidase Study Group. *JAMA* 2000; **283**: 1016–24.

Welliver R, Monto AS, Carewicz O *et al*. Effectiveness of oseltamivir in preventing influenza in household contact: a randomized controlled trial. *JAMA* 2001; **285**: 748–54.

8. Management

Immunization
Diagnosis
Standard treatment
Complications
The workplace

Immunization

In the early autumn of every year, all GPs in the UK initiate immunization programmes for influenza. Currently, UK government policy is to recommend influenza immunization for:

- all people aged 65 years and over
- people of all ages with chronic respiratory or heart disease, renal disease or diabetes mellitus
- all those who are immunocompromised
- all persons living in long-stay residential accommodation.

The question of whether to immunize a given individual rests entirely with the GP. However, targets are currently set by the government and monitored by the primary care organizations. In 2001, an overall nationwide target uptake of influenza immunization for individuals aged 65 years and above was set at 70%, with the aim of achieving a minimum uptake of 65%. The vaccine is given by intramuscular injection, and some vaccine recipients experience some local pain from this injection. There may also be some temporary soreness at the injection site that lasts 24–48 hours. Other side-effects are very rare, but include fever and muscle aches which can last up to two days.

It is impossible for influenza vaccine to cause influenza as it does not contain live virus – it contains only proteins derived from the virus. In some parts of the world the vaccine used contains intact but killed virus, which will also not cause influenza. The vaccine is contraindicated for people with severe allergy to hen's eggs, as the vaccine is manufactured in eggs and minute traces of egg protein may remain despite purification. Further information regarding vaccination on an annual basis is available on the Department of Health website (see Useful websites, p 53).

> It is impossible for influenza vaccine to cause influenza

The clinically compromised groups at special risk from influenza virus infection, who are therefore targeted for influenza vaccination, are outlined in Chapter 6. However, such is their importance that they are described more fully in Table 8.1.

Diagnosis

The clinical diagnosis of influenza virus infection is extremely difficult outside the influenza season, as many respiratory tract infections can mimic influenza. Even in the winter, if no clearcut epidemic is evident, the infection may be difficult to diagnose on clinical grounds alone. In general, an 'influenza-like illness' is recognized as an abrupt onset of fever and chills accompanied by:

- headache
- sore throat
- myalgias
- malaise
- anorexia
- dry cough.

The fever, which peaks within 24–48 hours of onset, can last from one to five days. Physical signs include:

- a hot and moist face
- flushing
- subconjunctival suffusion

Table 8.1
Risk groups for influenza immunization

General condition	Examples
Chronic respiratory disease, including asthma	Chronic obstructive pulmonary disease (COPD) Chronic bronchitis and emphysema Cystic fibrosis Interstitial lung fibrosis Pneumoconiosis Asthma requiring continuous or repeated use of inhaled or systemic steroids Asthma with previous exacerbations requiring hospital admission
Chronic heart disease	Chronic ischaemic heart disease Congenital heart disease and hypertensive heart disease requiring regular medication and follow-up (but excluding uncomplicated controlled hypertension) Chronic heart failure
Chronic renal disease	Nephrotic syndrome Chronic renal failure Renal transplantation patients
Diabetes	Diabetes mellitus requiring insulin or oral hypoglycaemic drugs
Immunosuppression	Occurring due to disease or treatment, including systemic steroids equivalent to 20 mg prednisolone daily for more than two weeks (Some immunocompromised patients may have a suboptimal immunological response to the vaccine)

Derived from Department of Health. Current vaccine and immunization issues 2001, P/L/CMO/2001/1.

- reddened nasal and mucosal surfaces
- clear nasal discharge.

In addition, adults occasionally have arthralgia, abdominal pain, chest pain and cervical lymphadenopathy. Children may also present with the features of a nonspecific febrile illness, or with a respiratory illness such as croup, bronchiolitis or bronchitis. These are very similar to the diseases caused by the parainfluenza viruses and respiratory syncytial virus (RSV).

During the influenza season (December–March), baseline rates of influenza can rise from below 50 cases to between 50 and 400 cases per 100 000 individuals each week. An influenza epidemic is defined as more than 400 cases per 100 000 of the population per week. Figure 1.4 shows the pattern of influenza activity in the UK over the past 12 years.

In practice, it is impossible for GPs to distinguish influenza virus infection from other respiratory tract infections, with certainty, on clinical grounds alone. Influenza viruses account for only about one-half of the influenza-like illness seen by GPs during the influenza season; the other pathogens involved being RSV, parainfluenza viruses, some picornaviruses and *Mycoplasma pneumoniae*. Although 'near patient testing' technologies are being developed, these currently lack the required sensitivity and specificity necessary for widespread deployment. Near patient testing involves beside tests that do not require samples to be sent to the laboratory. Therefore GPs are still required to make a diagnosis on purely clinical grounds, and in the absence of laboratory confirmation, this diagnosis is as an influenza-like illness.

Laboratory diagnosis is not normally carried out on a routine basis. At the start of the influenza season, as cases of influenza-like illness begin to appear in a community, the Public Health Laboratory Service (PHLS) is involved in confirming the infection as influenza in a small proportion of these initial 'index' cases. This is not only to register the presence and activity of the virus in the area, but also to determine if the circulating virus is a Type A or Type B virus. If it is a Type A virus, it is important to know whether it is an H3N2 or H1N1 subtype.

Laboratory diagnosis

As indicated above, not until near-patient testing technology becomes routine practice will it become possible to distinguish clinical influenza from the influenza-like illnesses with certainty. Nevertheless, during the influenza season, and in the presence of both a confirmed epidemic in the country and laboratory-confirmed cases of influenza in the community, an individual experiencing an abrupt onset of respiratory tract symptoms accompanied by malaise, headache, myalgia in the back and limbs and a temperature of 38–40°C, could be presumptively diagnosed as suffering from an influenza virus infection.

Although laboratory diagnosis is not normally sought for most cases of influenza, if hospitalization of a patient with suspected influenza infection becomes necessary, the infection must be diagnosed by the laboratory. In practice, the presence of the virus is best confirmed using nasopharyngeal aspirates. These may be collected using suction and trap methods in the hospital laboratory. In the doctor's surgery, throat swabs or preferably nasal washings may be taken if nasopharyngeal aspirates cannot be obtained. Throat swabs are, in general, not as effective as nasal washings for laboratory diagnosis of influenza. All samples for laboratory diagnosis must be placed into appropriate virus-preserving fluid medium, stored (for the minimum time possible) at 4°C and transported to the laboratory on ice as quickly as possible. Routine methods of laboratory testing for influenza virus include:

- examination for specific viral antigens by fluorescent microscopy
- cultivation of the virus in embryonated hen's eggs
- occasional cultivation of the virus in tissue culture.

> Nasal washes are more effective than throat swabs in the diagnosis of influenza in the laboratory

Diagnostic technologies for influenza virus which are still at the experimental stage and not yet available for routine use include the polymerase chain reaction (PCR) to specifically detect the viral nucleic acid.

Blood samples are usually taken at the onset of illness. However, the laboratory diagnosis of influenza virus infection can only be made on collection of a second blood sample from the patient at convalescence. Both samples are tested simultaneously to demonstrate a significant rise in the level of specific antibodies to the influenza virus in the convalescent sample. Such laboratory diagnosis is necessarily retrospective and is therefore of epidemiological rather than clinical significance.

Standard treatment

The management of influenza in individual patients entails both symptomatic treatment and the use of the novel antiviral agents that are becoming increasingly available. All patients with influenza should be encouraged to:

- drink adequate fluids
- take paracetamol to reduce symptoms
- stay off work
- rest at home in bed.

The nature and mechanisms of action of the antiviral agents operating against influenza are dealt with in Chapter 7. In practice, the neuraminidase inhibitors, which include zanamivir and oseltamivir, are the only drugs that can modify the natural history of influenza virus infection without causing unacceptable side-effects. The National Institute for Clinical Excellence (NICE) has provided guidance on the use of zanamivir in the treatment of influenza. On the basis that severe morbidity is uncommon in otherwise healthy adults suffering from influenza, zanamivir is not currently recommended in the UK for use in this group. However, the results of further studies are awaited.

Zanamivir and oseltamivir act against a stage of the virus replication cycle (release of virus from the infected cell) that is specific to the influenza viruses. Therefore, they have no beneficial activity against other viruses or against *Mycoplasma pneumoniae*. There are also no harmful effects of these antiviral drugs should they be given to individuals suffering from an influenza-like illness.

> Patients with influenza should be encouraged to drink adequate fluids, to take paracetamol to reduce symptoms, to stay off work and to rest at home in bed

As soon as the PHLS has signalled that influenza is circulating in the community, it is recommended that zanamivir is prescribed for 'at risk' adults who present within 36 hours of the onset of an influenza-like illness, and who are able to commence treatment within 48 hours of the onset of these symptoms. The 'at risk' adults are individuals falling into one or more of the categories listed in Table 6.1.

Treatment with zanamivir consists of a five-day course of 10 mg of the drug given twice daily by inhalation via a Diskhaler device. At the time of writing, the NHS cost of zanamivir is £24 per five-day course of treatment. The frail elderly might have difficulty both in handling the Diskhaler device and in manipulating it, and may require help with the inhalations. It is envisaged that oral treatments with oseltamivir will be available in the near future. Extensive guidance on the use of zanamivir in patients can be found on the NICE and the Department of Health websites.

> The neuraminidase inhibitors are the only drugs that can modify the natural history of influenza virus infection without causing unacceptable side-effects

Complications

Pneumonia

The most common serious complication of influenza is pneumonia, and this may occur at the same time as the influenza-like illness or could arise up to two weeks afterwards.

- If the pneumonia appears during the influenza-like illness, then it is possible that it is a primary viral pneumonia caused by the virus itself. However, this is relatively uncommon.
- If the pneumonia commences after apparent recovery from the influenza infection, then it is most likely that there is a bacterial superinfection. This is usually due to either *Streptococcus pneumoniae* or *Staphylococcus aureus*.

All influenza virus pneumonias should be assumed to be bacterial because of the high mortality rate, particularly in the 'at risk' groups. All patients should, therefore, be carefully evaluated for symptoms and signs of pneumonia. Any patient with evidence of lung consolidation should be evaluated for possible hospital admission and should be treated with antibiotics using the guidance supplied by the British Thoracic Society. This would include the use of aminopenicillin and/or an oral macrolide (such as erythromycin). It is common practice to include the use of oral flucloxacillin in patients who present with pneumonia after influenza, because of the increased frequency of *Staphylococcus aureus* pneumonias in this group.

GPs will advise patients with influenza to stay at home, but should remain aware of the possibility of complications arising in the patient, eg pneumonia. GPs are faced with the tension of coping with an unmanageable home-visiting load and missing a pneumonia. It is important that the physician can advise the patient with influenza to be aware of symptoms such as:

- shortness of breath
- pleuritic chest pain
- haemoptysis.

Any or all of these may herald the development of a pneumonia. Should such symptoms arise in the patient, he or she should contact the doctor immediately.

Residential care homes

If a GP encounters a cluster of influenza-like illnesses in a nursing home or other residential facility, the initial cases should be treated as outlined above. The most important intervention is to contact the local consultant in communicable disease control. Subsequently, the public health authorities will be able to make an assessment of the risk to other residents, and institute control of infection policies, such as chemoprophylaxis, if necessary.

Bacterial infections

The complications that may follow influenza virus infection in an elderly individual, in an individual suffering from a chronic respiratory or cardiovascular condition, or very occasionally in a healthy adult, are likely to be more severe than any complications that may follow an influenza-like illness. This is due not only to the almost complete destruction of the ciliated epithelial cells lining the trachea and bronchii of the respiratory tract, but is also associated with the systemic symptoms arising during influenza virus infection that, although not fully understood, seem to impose a considerable strain on the body. This interaction of the influenza virus with the host can be considerably more severe than that caused by other infectious agents that give rise to influenza-like illnesses.

However, there could be complications following infection with *Mycoplasma pneumoniae*. Infection by this agent may result in a lengthy illness sometimes accompanied by clinical depression and occasional haematological and neurological sequelae. This distinguishes infection by *Mycoplasma pneumoniae* from an influenza infection with complications.

There are few serious complications subsequent to RSV infection in adults, and infections by the parainfluenza virus are usually mild. In infants and young children ≤ two years of age (a group not normally victims of disease caused by the influenza virus), RSV can cause a severe, acute bronchiolitis that carries a mortality rate of 0.1% in untreated cases. The parainfluenza viruses are associated with croup (an acute laryngotracheobronchitis) in children under five years of age, although this infection carries no significant mortality.

The workplace

Management of influenza in the workplace centres around vaccination. When faced with an impending epidemic, some industrial companies may choose to offer their employees immunization with the current vaccine, in order to minimize sickness and absenteeism through influenza or influenza-like illness. In the special case of the essential service industries – such as the healthcare professions, the fire and police services – immunization is recommended. This is especially true where advance notice has been received of the arrival of an influenza Type A or B strain that has significant antigenic differences from preceding strains.

It must be stressed that influenza vaccination in the UK remains optional. It is at the discretion of the individual to receive the injection, and at the discretion of the commercial or industrial company to offer it.

Further reading

Boivin G, Osterhaus AD, Gaudreau A et al. Role of picornaviruses in flu-like illnesses of adults enrolled in an oseltamivir treatment study who had no evidence of influenza virus infection. *J Clin Microbiol* 2002; **40**: 330–4.

Furey A, Robinson E, Young Y. Improving immunisation coverage in 2000–2001: A baseline survey, review of the evidence and sharing of best practice. *Commun Dis Public Health* 2001; **4**: 183–7.

Gupta A, Morris G, Thomas P, Hasan M. Influenza vaccination coverage in old people's homes in Carmarthenshire, UK, during the winter of 1998/99. *Vaccine* 2000; **18**: 2471–5.

Gupta A, Makinde K, Morris G et al. Influenza immunisation coverage in older hospitalised patients during winter 1998–99 in Carmarthenshire, UK. *Age Ageing*; **29**: 211–13.

Kumpulainen V, Makela M. Influenza among healthy employees: a cost-benefit analysis. *Scand J Infect Dis* 1997; **29**: 181–5.

Useful websites

Association of Medical Microbiologists

www.amm.co.uk/pubs/fa_influenza
[The Association of Medical Microbiologist's website comprises three pages of basic facts about the influenza viruses and their transmission, together with a description of the clinical syndrome of influenza, its prevention and treatment]

Department of Health

www.doh.gov.uk
[A generally useful website with regularly updated information on topical issues and a number of links to the NHS]
www.doh.gov.uk/zanamivirguidance
[This website is designed specifically to provide up-to-date information on the anti-influenza drug zanamivir, and it is primarily aimed at the general practitioner. There is guidance on the conditions under which zanamivir can be used, sections concerned with both national and local action and links to sites covering patient management not dealt with by the NICE recommendations for treatment of influenza]

European Scientific Working Group on influenza

www.eswi.org/intro.cfm
[A new website from the European Scientific Working Group on Influenza that offers updated information on influenza viruses, the disease, diagnosis, epidemiology, prevention and control. The group also issues a twice-yearly bulletin, 'Influenza', available on the website]

'Flu index page

www.phls.co.uk/facts/influenza/flu.htm
[A website from the Public Health Laboratory Services specifically concerned with accessing up-to-date information about most aspects of influenza, including 'frequently asked questions on flu', the current situation on influenza surveillance, the treatment of influenza and PHLS publications on influenza. There is also a link to related influenza websites]

Influenza vaccination

www.jr2.ox.ac.uk/bandolier/band73/b73-7.html
[Summarizes the findings of recent clinical trials of influenza vaccines in terms of their efficacy and any documented adverse effects. Provides information on the value and effectiveness of influenza vaccines]

Morbidity statistics

www.rcgp-bru.demon.co.uk
[The Royal College of General Practitioners website provides weekly morbidity statistics on respiratory and influenza-like illness from general practices, as well as the results of statistical analyses on consulting patterns, age group differences and comparisons between current and previous years with respect to the incidence of influenza]

National Institute for Clinical Excellence

www.nice.org.uk/nice-web/
[A comprehensive website providing a valuable starting point for accessing updated information about recent advances in the treatment of

diseases, including influenza. The website also includes general information about NICE and its activities along with link to further websites on influenza]

World Health Organization

www.who.int/emc/diseases/flu/index
[A World Health Organization website that covers, through many links, basic facts about influenza, the WHO influenza programme, national pandemic preparation plans, recommendations for vaccine composition and the use of vaccines and other preventative measures. For the influenza fanatic there is also a link to the 'Influenza Bibliography listings', which lists all publications worldwide that touch upon the virus, the infection and its control]

Index

Page numbers in *italics* refer to information that is shown only in a table or diagram.

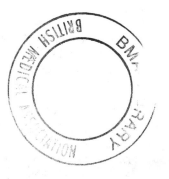

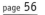